DAVID ZINCZENKO

with *Michael Freidson*

ZERO BELLY

BREAKFASTS

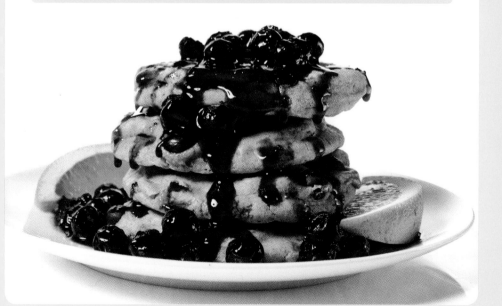

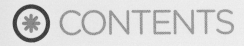# CONTENTS

WAKE UP SLIMMER EVERY DAY!

What if I told you that you could eat pancakes and waffles, chocolate cereal and egg sandwiches, omelets and breakfast burritos—and lose up to 16 pounds in 14 days? You can with *Zero Belly Breakfasts*. They'll have you looking and feeling great in no time flat, thanks to hundreds of delicious and nutritious breakfast secrets—and more than 100 mouthwatering recipes you can prepare in minutes!

I know because I've seen it happen.

INTRODUCTION ✱

In 2015, I shared *Zero Belly Diet* with a test panel of more than 500 people, some of whom lost as much as 16 pounds in just 14 days, and up to 3 inches off their waist. June Caron, 57, lost 12 pounds in 2 weeks and 4 dress sizes in 1 year. "Hail to the Chef," she said of the recipes. "My confidence is up, my happiness is up!" Fred Sparks, 39, lost 21 pounds and 5 inches off his waist in 6 weeks. "I met a group of co-workers who hasn't seen me in a month," he shared, "and they were all astonished."

The secret to the plan is the new science of nutritional genetics, the study of how our genes are turned on and off by the foods we eat. Simply making a handful of tweaks to your diet and lifestyle can help improve your gut health, dampen inflammation, turn off your fat genes, and start your body shedding fat—in particular, belly fat—almost automatically.

You see, some foods turn our fat genes "on"—causing seemingly irreversible weight gain. That's why some of us stay thin and why some of us can't lose weight no matter how hard we try. With *Zero Belly Breakfasts*, you'll eat power foods that act directly on those switches, turning them to "off" and allowing for easy, rapid, and sustainable weight loss. These foods also help heal your digestive system, keeping those gene switches turned off and setting you up for a lifetime of leanness.

And every single *Zero Belly Breakfasts* recipe is made with these fat-blasting foods.

What's So Special About Breakfast?

What isn't? The old adage that it's the "most important meal of the day" has been proven time and again, most recently by the American Heart Association, which just changed their guidelines to indicate that eating earlier in the day can lead to a healthier heart, staving off cardiac arrests and strokes. "When we eat may be important to consider, in addition to what we eat," said Marie-Pierre St-Onge of Columbia University Medical Center in New York, who led the team that wrote the guidelines. The research team found that the body processes sugars better during the day than at night.

INTRODUCTION ✳

And yet more than 30 percent of us skip breakfast. And that's partially why Americans are sick and fat. More than one-third of us are obese. An estimated 86 million of us have prediabetes. Health care costs are at an all-time high—and 85 percent of us have seen a doctor in the last year (at an average cost of $740 a pop).

I wrote the Zero Belly series because I know many of you are sick and tired of your health care system, in addition to being sick and tired. Zero Belly Breakfasts aren't just delicious ways to start every morning, but a prescription for a leaner, fitter, healthier you.

Each of the book's 100-plus recipes features fat-burning proteins, belly-filling fibers, and healthy fats that will boost your metabolism and lead to all-day (and night!) weight loss. As a result, you'll:

> Lose up to 16 pounds in 14 days.

> Melt away stubborn fat, from your belly first.

> Put an end to bloating and discomfort.

> Detox from unhealthy foods so you can enjoy all-day energy.

> Turn off your fat storage genes and make long-term weight loss effortless.

> Look and feel younger and healthier than ever!

It Worked for Them!

Other diets can help you lose weight, but only *Zero Belly Breakfasts* attacks fat on a genetic level, placing a bull's-eye on the fat cells that matter most: visceral fat, the type of fat ensconced in your belly. These fat cells act like an invading army, increasing inflammation and putting you at risk for diabetes, Alzheimer's, arthritis, heart disease, and cancer. Visceral fat can also alter your hormone levels, erode muscle tissue, increase your chances of depression, and destroy your sex drive. But you can turn the odds in your favor.

The Zero Belly series shows you how to deactivate your fat genes, rev up your metabolism, banish bloat, and balance your digestive health, allowing you to easily build lean, strong stomach muscle and strip away unwanted belly fat without sacrificing calories or spending hours at the gym. The result: weight loss that is easier, faster, more lasting, and more delicious than you'd ever imagine.

I was stunned and inspired by the results of that amazing 500-person test panel. It was made up of men and women who agreed to send us weekly reports of their experience. They told us that they lost weight quickly and with ease following the Zero Belly Diet. Here are just some of their results from the first 14 days:

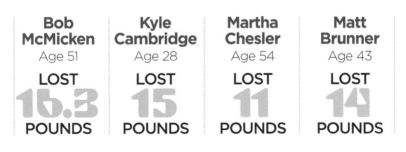

Bob McMicken	Kyle Cambridge	Martha Chesler	Matt Brunner
Age 51	Age 28	Age 54	Age 43
LOST	LOST	LOST	LOST
16.3	15	11	14
POUNDS	POUNDS	POUNDS	POUNDS

INTRODUCTION ✳

And It'll Work for You!

By eating Zero Belly Breakfasts, and following Zero Belly Diet, you will lose the weight you want—each one is not just low in calories but nearly void of added sugars, on the cutting edge of the latest governmental guidelines.

In fact, for the first time ever, the USDA has issued guidelines recommending that Americans keep their consumption of added sugars low—to no more than 10 percent of overall calories, or about 180 calories a day for women and 200 for men.

That means 45 grams of sugar a day, tops, or about eleven teaspoons. And organizations from the American Heart Association to the World Health Organization recommend cutting that number further; they say no more than 25 grams of added sugar a day—about six sugar packets—is best for optimal health.

Chances are, you're eating four, five, or even six times that.

Every one of the Zero Belly Breakfasts is calibrated to keep you well below that amount. If you needed a wake-up call, consider yourself "woke." Regardless of your health history, your lifestyle, or even your genes, *Zero Belly Breakfasts* will give you the power to flatten your belly, heal your body, soothe your soul, and wake up happier than ever!

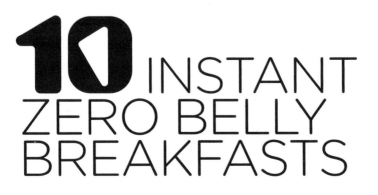

10 INSTANT ZERO BELLY BREAKFASTS

1

Simmer a cup of sugar-free tomato sauce in a skillet. Crack eggs directly into the sauce and swirl in the whites, while leaving the yolks untouched. Cook until the whites are firm and the yolk is set but still runny. Top with lots of cracked black pepper and fresh parsley, if you like.

2

Combine cooked quinoa in a pan with ½ cup of almond milk, 1 tablespoon of extra-virgin olive oil,

golden raisins, a touch of brown sugar, and toasted walnuts. Heat until hot and creamy.

3

Add salsa and grated Daiya cheese to a small oven-safe bowl or ramekin. Crack 2 eggs over the top and bake in a 400°F oven for 10 to 12 minutes, until the whites are just set.

4

Spread a toasted gluten-free English muffin with almond butter. Top with sliced bananas, a drizzle of agave syrup, and crushed almonds.

5

Stir a spoonful of peanut butter into a bowl of plain instant oatmeal. Top with diced apples, crushed walnuts, and a touch of agave syrup.

6

Denver scramble: Sauté chunks of ham, sliced mushrooms, onions, and bell pepper in a large nonstick sauté pan until the vegetables are soft and lightly browned. Add beaten eggs and scramble until the eggs are nearly set.

7

Scramble eggs gently over low heat. Stir in

pieces of broken tortillas, canned roasted chilies, and diced tomatoes. Season with salt, pepper, and a few shakes of hot sauce.

8

Heat 1 cup of spicy, not-too-chunky salsa in a skillet. Add a few handfuls of tortilla chips and an egg.

9

Sauté an egg in extra-virgin olive oil. Slide on top of a bowl of gluten-free spaghetti with extra-virgin olive oil and crushed red pepper flakes.

10

Roast or blanch 7 asparagus spears until tender. Arrange 4 or 5 on a plate, top with sunny-side up eggs.

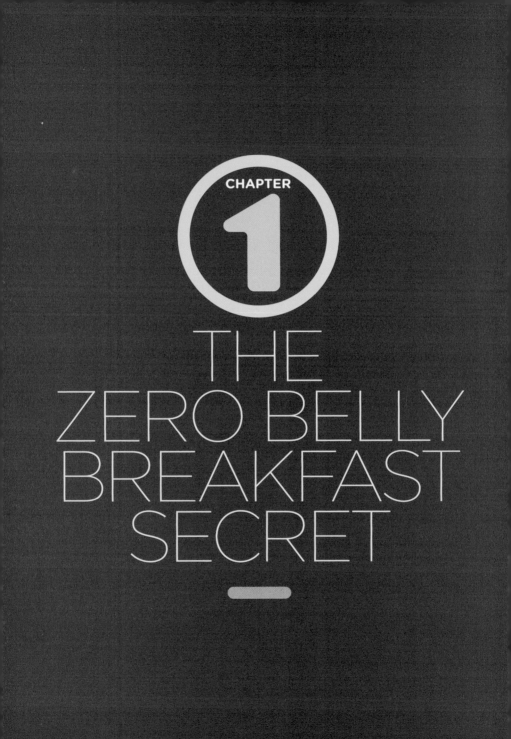

Griddle cakes with freshly tapped maple syrup; fluffy scrambled eggs with cracked pepper and a fresh tomato; crunchy grits with whole milk and a biscuit; eggs Benedict and a Bloody Mary; the classic egg and bacon sandwich, made with crispy rashers; creamy Greek yogurt topped with fresh berries and dark chocolate.

Some people wake up to seize the day. I wake up to eat breakfast.

It's my favorite meal of the day, and has been all my life—although my choices weren't always the healthiest. As a kid growing up in the 1980s, I greeted every morning with my BFFs (that's Breakfast Friends Forever): Cap'N Crunch, Count Chocula, and the Cookie Crook, literally pouring chocolate chip cookies into a bowl. By the time I was 14, I had a belly the size of my dad's, carrying 212 pounds on my 6-foot frame.

I wasn't alone.

The adult obesity rate has more than doubled since the 1980s, growing from 15 percent to 35 percent in the mid-2000s. It's now at 35.7 percent—yes, more than one-third of Americans are considered obese, according to the National Institutes of Health. Obesity shortened my father's life, and for most of my childhood I struggled with that extra 25 pounds as well. I figured it was my genetic destiny to be fat, too.

But like you, I got sick and tired of being sick and tired, and since then, I've made it my life's work to learn everything there is to know about belly fat.

As the editorial director of *Men's Health, Women's Health,* and *Prevention*, I poured over the latest research about obesity, weight loss, and a longer life. My findings helped inform *The Abs Diet*, and while there, I wrote *Eat This, Not That!*, the first of a bestselling series that helped Americans make the right food choice—every time—in a world before there were calorie counts on every menu. *Eat This, Not That!* went on to sell 8 million copies, and lives on at eatthis.com, the most authoritative website anywhere about weight loss and nutrition. But I still wanted to know how to blast belly fat—for good. And that's when I discovered that certain foods can target your belly specifically, especially if you eat them in the morning. That's when I knew I had to write the Zero Belly series.

Turn Off Your Fat Genes—with Zero Belly

We all want to look good in a bathing suit at the beach, but there's a far more important reason to lose that roll of belly fat creeping over your waistband: your health and longevity. Belly fat—or "visceral fat," as the doctors call it—is the common link in almost every major life-threatening disease we face today, from diabetes to heart disease, from dementia to cancer.

That's because visceral fat is like an invading army. It

tries to take over your body by releasing compounds that erode muscle, damage your ability to manage insulin, and increase the levels of inflammation in your body. These three things not only put you at risk for heart disease, diabetes, and Alzheimer's, but they do something else: They set you up for more belly fat.

By reducing the amount of belly fat you carry around, you will dramatically improve your chances of living a long and active life.

Easier said than done? Sure. Except that the new science of nutrigenetics—the study of how food and DNA interact—is making it easier than ever, and turning the odds of flat belly success in your favor. It's this exciting new field of research that forms the basis of Zero Belly, the first program to eliminate belly fat, not through traditional calorie-restrictive weight-loss methods but by actually "turning off" our fat genes, altering our genetic destiny, and reversing the march of obesity and its related diseases.

Since introducing the series, it's sold hundreds of thousands of copies and changed the lives of that many readers worldwide.

Because obesity is a worldwide epidemic. A study by Public Health England found that children there are eating half their daily allowance of sugar before they head to school. As a result, "a quarter of five-year-olds have tooth decay and nearly a fifth of children are already obese by the time they leave primary school," reports the BBC.

How Breakfast Targets Your Belly

The solution for this worldwide epidemic is clear. It's breakfast.

We've all heard the saying that breakfast is the most important meal of the day, but the author of that adage probably didn't have doughnuts and Belgian waffles in mind when they said it. With so many high-carb, high-sugar options available in the a.m., breakfast is often the cause of our low energy throughout the day as well as our expanding waistlines. Instead of reaching for a starchy snack that will give you a quick burst of energy and cause you to crash later, enjoying a meal that combines protein, healthy fats, and slow carbohydrates will help your energy levels stay stable all day and won't undo the hard work you've done to achieve your Zero Belly.

The studies prove they work. New research from universities around the world have come to the conclusion that eating a healthy, high-protein breakfast every day—like the kinds found in *Zero Belly Breakfasts*—leads to weight loss and prevents obesity.

In one, published in the *American Journal of Epidemiology,* scientists evaluated the relation between eating patterns and obesity, over a four-year period, for nearly 500 participants. They found those who ate regular meals throughout the day, including a consistent breakfast, lost more weight than those who didn't, while "skipping breakfast was associated with increased prevalence of obesity." (What's interesting was that where you eat breakfast also made a difference. Those researchers found that if you ate breakfast at home, you'd lose more weight.)

That's why *Zero Belly Breakfasts* is so important. The recipes contain a unique approach to weight loss that attacks belly fat in three ways.

FIRST, they light a fire under your metabolism, triggering your body's natural calorie-burning mechanism—a mechanism that specifically targets belly fat. *Zero Belly Breakfasts* unleash the power of protein, fiber, and healthy fats to burn calories by encouraging lean muscle growth and maximizing the thermogenic effects of eating—in effect, burning more calories by eating more great food.

SECOND, *Zero Belly Breakfasts* attack inflammation

throughout the body by triggering your digestive system's natural defense system, shrinking bloat, easing digestion, and flattening your stomach with shocking rapidity. While the diet plan isn't strictly dairy-free or gluten-free, these meals substantially reduce your intake of lactose (the naturally occurring sugar in dairy), gluten (the protein found in wheat), and animal-derived saturated fat, and they will eliminate inflammation-causing additives.

THIRD, this program turns off your fat-storage genes by focusing on nine power food groups that are linked directly to the emerging science of how nutrients in food influence gene expression.

And these breakfasts are simple to make, with ingredients you already have at home. To wit:

- A study published in *Plant Foods for Human Nutrition* found that eating oatmeal aided in weight loss, improved liver function, and got hip-to-waist ratio into a more desirable territory.

- Scrambled eggs are one of the easiest ways to enjoy a protein-packed breakfast without a ton of preparation. A study by the *International Journal of Obesity* found that consuming eggs at breakfast helped participants lose 65 percent more weight.

- Protein-rich quinoa provides a nutty, slightly crunchy texture that works well with the soft sweetness of berries, bananas, and baked apples.

Other cookbooks can help you lose weight, but only *Zero Belly Breakfasts* places a bull's-eye on the fat cells that matter most. The result: weight loss that is easier, faster, more lasting, and more delicious than you'd ever imagine.

FOUR WAYS BREAKFAST IS BEST

Enjoying a delicious Zero Belly breakfast every morning will help you quickly strip away flab in a number of ways. Here's what makes *Zero Belly Breakfasts* so effective:

1 They Help You Keep the Weight Off

Science proved it. Of people who've lost 30 pounds or more, 80 percent kept the weight off by eating a high-protein breakfast every day, according to a study done by the National Weight Control Registry, who concluded that "eating breakfast is a characteristic common to successful weight loss maintainers."

2 They Help You Eat Less

A study in *Obesity* found that eating a high-protein breakfast led to "the prevention of body fat gain, voluntary reductions in daily intake, and reductions in daily hunger." Meanwhile, skipping it leads to eating more food throughout the day—and unnecessary weight around your midsection.

3 They're the Most Important Meal of the Day—for Fat Burn

Your mom was right. "People who eat their largest daily meal at breakfast are far more likely to lose weight and waist line circumference than those who eat a large dinner," reported researchers in a 2013 study from Tel Aviv University titled "Eating a Big Breakfast Fights Obesity and Disease." "They also had significantly lower levels of insulin, glucose, and triglycerides throughout the day, translating into a lower risk of cardiovascular disease, diabetes, hypertension, and high cholesterol."

4 They Taste Amazing!

And you won't believe how hearty they are. For example, steak and eggs may seem like a rich combo, but they can also be a part of your quest to banish belly fat, thanks to the high protein content of this satisfying meal. Choose a lean cut of meat and you can enjoy this low-carb breakfast without concerns over its heart-healthiness.

Regardless of your health history, your lifestyle, or even your genes, *Zero Belly Breakfasts* will give you the power to flatten your belly, heal your body, soothe your soul, and wake up happier than ever!

YOUR ZERO BELLY CHEAT SHEET

"Crazy busy." There's no escape from it. No matter who you ask—family, friends, colleagues, retirees—everybody seems to be "crazy busy." You're crazy busy, too. That's why we made *Zero Belly Diet* easy to follow and simple to practice. If you're new to the program, here's an at-a-glance guide to the Zero Belly principles, the diet plan that will flatten your belly, turn off your fat genes, and help keep you lean for life. (And if you would like a turbo-charged version of the program, check out the "Zero Belly BreakFAST" chapter!)

SUBJECT: Number of Meals

GUIDELINE: Three meals, one snack, and one Zero Belly Smoothie per day.

SUBJECT: The ZERO BELLY Foods

GUIDELINE: Each of the meals and snacks is built around the 9 ZERO BELLY Foods, each carefully selected for its micronutrient content. Every meal or snack should have protein, fiber, and healthy fat, derived from one of these sources:

Zero Belly Smoothies

Eggs

Red fruits

Olive oil and other healthy fats

Beans, rice, oats, and other healthy fiber

Extra plant protein

Leafy greens, green tea, and bright vegetables

Lean meats and fish

Your favorite spices and flavors (ginger, cinnamon, even chocolate)

SUBJECT: Portion Size

GUIDELINE: While most diets center around controlling calorie intake, Zero Belly focuses on maximizing your intake of key nutrients. When you eat protein, fiber, and healthy fat, you'll crowd much of the junk out of your diet and control your hunger and calorie intake naturally.

SUBJECT: Secret Weapons

GUIDELINE: Smoothies. You'll find some in this book, and 100+ more in *Zero Belly Smoothies,* and it's in these delicious drinks that the principles of Zero Belly come together so brilliantly. Each of the smoothie recipes combine the Zero Belly Foods into high-nutrient meals that are ready in just 90 seconds, and each combines protein, fiber, and healthy fat to ensure you're always highly fueled and never hungry.

SUBJECT: Nutritional Ingredients to Emphasize

GUIDELINE: Protein, fiber, healthy fats

SUBJECT: Nutritional Ingredients to Limit

GUIDELINE: Dairy, wheat gluten, added sugars. (Note: Zero Belly is not strictly dairy-free or gluten-free. But because these can cause bloating and inflammation in some people, I've made sure that the entire program can be done without either ingredient. Each of the recipes in this book is gluten-free and dairy-free.)

SUBJECT: Alcohol

GUIDELINE: Limit yourself to no more than two or three drinks per week to maximize the benefits of the program. Because of its high concentration of resveratrol, a compound that helps turn off fat-storage genes, red wine is the best choice

SUBJECT: Exercise Program

GUIDELINE: To turbocharge the weight-loss effects of Zero Belly, I've created the Zero Belly Workouts, a unique full-body fitness experience that builds abs while simultaneously toning your entire body. The complete Zero Belly Workout plan is found in *Zero Belly Diet*.

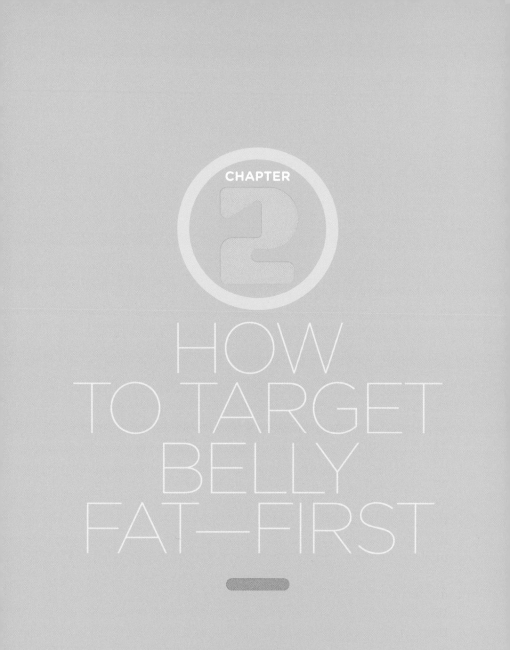

CHAPTER

2

HOW TO TARGET BELLY FAT—FIRST

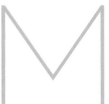organ Minor was fed up.

The 24-year-old firefighter from Coalinga, California, had been gaining weight steadily for several years, and one day she hit 196 pounds. She didn't like the way she looked, and she didn't like the way the extra weight made her feel, especially on the job—where her fitness could literally make the difference between life and death. "I was gaining weight like crazy, and I decided I was tired of it and it was time to make a change," Morgan told us. "So I started exercising."

Adopting a serious fitness regimen made a huge difference—within 9 months she'd gotten down to a healthy 160. But then her weight loss plateaued, and she realized that exercise alone wasn't going to get her to her goals. "I started looking for a good diet to incorporate with my work-outs to get this last bit of stubborn flab off." Then she found *Zero Belly Diet*, and the speed with which she lost the last 11 pounds—and uncovered her abs—astonished her.

Within a week she had dropped 7 pounds, and after just 21 days, a sculpted stomach emerged—Morgan had shed four inches off her waist. "I had plateaued at 160 for over a month, and Zero Belly helped me lose more than ten pounds in 3 weeks!"

Now it's your turn.

Zero Belly Breakfasts are made using the same principles that helped Morgan—and thousands of others—drop those stubborn pounds. These delicious recipes—each of them gluten-free, lactose-free, and packed with amazing flavor—combine the magic of cooking at home with the metabolism turbocharge of our handpicked, insanely healthy superfoods. Each one also addresses the three Zero Belly questions:

WHERE'S MY PROTEIN?
WHERE'S MY FIBER?
WHERE'S MY HEALTHY FAT?

Zero Belly Breakfasts are perfectly calibrated to have all three—and as a result, you'll never crave fatty foods or feel bad again.

The first thing Morgan noticed was that on Zero Belly, she didn't have to feel hungry all the time. "I don't feel like I'm dieting," she said, even as she was losing a pound a day in the first week. The reason: Eating the right foods controls hunger. In fact, researchers have found that a diet high in unhealthy fats modified the way leptin—the "satiety" hormone that's produced by our fat cells—behaves inside the body. Other studies have shown that our fat-storage genes are turned "on" by inflammation—and sugar and unhealthy fats are the biggest culprits. But you can reduce inflammation (and hunger) and shed flab by eating more of the right foods: red fruits, leafy greens and colorful vegetables, high-fiber carbs and healthy fats and proteins—three meals a day, plus a snack.

Zero Belly worked for Bob McMicken, too.

A hardworking food service director and father of

seven, he knows stress. The 51-year-old Lancaster, California, resident was toting around 229 pounds, much of it balanced dangerously along his waistline, and he knew his health was a major concern. Sick of feeling bloated and emotionally drained, Bob made a commitment to take control of his health and signed up for the Zero Belly Test Panel. Within days of following the easy menu, Bob's bloat seemed to disappear.

In fact, in just two weeks, Bob lost a stunning 16.3 pounds. And in less than six weeks, he lost 24 pounds and saw his waist size drop from 39 inches to 33 inches. "I found my favorite shirt finally covered my belly again!"

"Before Zero Belly I felt bloated, fat, and depressed," he says. "Now I feel better, have more energy, and am smiling!"

Here's how Zero Belly Breakfasts will work for you:

They're Powered by Protein

It burns fat. It builds muscle. And it tastes awesome. It's easy to love protein. All of our favorite foods—burgers, steaks, pork chops, bacon—are packed with it. That's why you should be eating more of it before noon.

"There is new research emerging on protein at breakfast and its effect on weight," says Angela Lemond, a registered dietitian in Texas. "Getting adequate protein at breakfast can help with overall satiety throughout the day." It'll also prevent a sugar crash. A new study in the *Journal of Nutrition* found that participants who ate more protein at breakfast had more stable blood sugar levels, important news for diabetics and anyone looking to avoid a post-lunch slump.

And with the ever-growing popularity of whey-protein shakes, we're taking in more of this essential muscle maker than ever before.

But are we eating the right kind? While that $9 whey smoothie might be helping your weight loss, there are far more effective—and less expensive—choices. In fact, new research indicates that if you want to lose weight, more of your protein should come not from meat and dairy but from vegetables. In a study earlier this year in the *Journal of Diabetes Investigation*, researchers discovered that patients who ingested higher amounts of vegetable protein were far less susceptible to obesity, diabetes, and heart disease than those who got most of their protein from animal sources. And a second study in *Nutrition Journal* found that "plant protein intakes may play a role in preventing obesity."

Although not a vegetarian diet, Zero Belly heavily features plant- and egg-based proteins—all Zero Belly Smoothies are vegan—with plenty of meat for you carnivores, too.

They Boost Your Gut Bacteria

The secret to solving your health and weight issues aren't just cutting calories, exercising, and drinking less Coke. It's also making sure you eat more bugs.

No, we're not talking about those bugs. We're talking about the trillions of helpful bacteria that live in your gut and play a fundamental role in maintaining a healthy and happy body. (And yes, we said trillions—many estimates equate that number with making up three pounds of your total body weight!) This community, referred to by scientists as your "gut microbiota" or "gut microbiome," can be composed of around 500 species that each supply their own benefits: Some of them break down your food and extract nutrients; others hunt for food pathogens; and others help protect you from colds and flus. In fact, they play such a critical role in our health that many experts have started to refer to the microbiome as its own organ. All of this sounds like a good thing—so what's the problem?

The problem is this: When we eat too much junk food (especially sugar) and take too many drugs (like antibiotics or antidepressants), we can knock our digestive systems out of whack and disrupt the composition of our gut. When your good gut bugs are depleted, bad bacteria can take over, causing health issues that range from skin conditions to depression. What's more, researchers are finding that obese people have different gut bugs than healthy-weight people, suggesting that cultivating a proper gut garden may help solve weight troubles.

So, if you're struggling with weight loss, anxiety, stress, skin issues, fatigue, or chronic sickness, you might want to start looking at your gut.

The good news is that you can empower your gut microbiota and help it fight back against the invaders by feeding your beneficial bacteria the foods they—and you—need to stay healthy.

Each Zero Belly Breakfast is designed to go easy on your gut.

They Keep You Fuller, Longer

What you eat after rolling out of bed has the power to banish cravings, turbocharge energy, and keep your waistline in check—all day long. Breakfast munchers eat 12 percent healthier throughout the day, according to data from the app Eatery, which tracks users' daily chow-down habits. "Skipping breakfast makes you more likely to overindulge at your next meal, or eat mid-morning snacks that are high in calories and sugar to ward off hunger until lunch," says Amari Cheffer, RD. With more than 20 grams of protein each, Zero Belly Breakfasts will keep you full until noon.

They Put You in Charge

Here's a little secret that the restaurant industry doesn't want you to know: The absolute best recipe for a flat belly is . . . any recipe. As long as you're the one doing the cooking.

In a study in the journal *Public Health Nutrition,* people who ate at a restaurant on any given day took in an additional 200 calories more than those who prepared all their own meals. Even if you eat just one meal a day from a restaurant, that's enough to add 21 pounds of body weight every year.

In fact, cooking at home regularly is so good for you that it helps you eat less even on nights when you do go out to a restaurant—probably because you've become used to serving yourself sane portion sizes instead of the mind-bending, monster-size entrées most restaurants dish out!

They Are Easy—and Fun— to Make!

Indulge in the 100+ recipes in this book—or combine the Zero Belly superfoods to make your own.

KITCHEN SECRET

BALL MASON JARS

What do Mason jar salads, overnight oats, and omelets in a jar have in common? They're all über healthy, hip—and require Mason jars to be made. To get in on this good-for-you trend, pick up a big pack of jars, which come 12 to a pack. Aside from their culinary uses, they make great storage solutions for odds and ends, or for your Zero Belly spices.

THE ZERO BELLY FOODS

This book doesn't contain the complete Zero Belly Diet, but every recipe is made with at least one of the key Zero Belly Diet foods. In this excerpt from *Zero Belly Cookbook,* you'll learn how each one leads to maximum fat burn and a healthier, happier you.

ZERO BELLY SMOOTHIES
Maximize Nutritional Intake

To experience the full impact of the Zero Belly program, each day you should supplement your regular meals with one of the blended smoothie drinks you'll find starting on page 208. These drinks are so delicious, and so easy to make, that you can have them for breakfast, as a snack, as a meal replacement, or even as a dessert. Studies show that high-protein, low-fat smoothies are highly effective at rushing nutrients into your body, particularly your muscles.

I've stripped all the Zero Belly Smoothie recipes of the dairy, added sugars, and artificial ingredients so common in popular commercial shakes, and packed them with real fruits, nuts, vegan proteins, and dairy alternatives such as almond milk and coconut milk. Why the alternative milks? First, dairy can be difficult to digest for some folks—and poor digestion leads to inflammation, which leads to weight gain. But there's more to it than that: In 2014, Swedish scientists at Uppsala University found that women who drank three or more glasses of milk a day died at nearly twice the rate of those who drank less than one glass a day. Broken bones were more common in women who were heavy milk drinkers as well. While this is only a preliminary study, it's further reason why using nondairy milk in your daily smoothie is a wise move.

EGGS
Turn Off Visceral Fat Genes

Eggs are the single best dietary source of the B vitamin choline, an essential nutrient used in the construction of all of the body's cell membranes. Choline deficiency is linked directly to the genes that cause visceral fat accumulation, particularly in the liver. Yet according to a 2015 National Health and Nutrition Examination Survey, only a small percentage of all Americans eat daily diets that meet the U.S. Institute of Medicine's Adequate Intake of 425 mg for women and 550 mg for men.

RED FRUIT
Turn Off Obesity Genes

Like professional basketball players, all fruits are good at what they do. But a red hue is a sign that your snack is just that little bit better—watermelon is to honeydew what LeBron is to a backup on the Knicks. And since the release of *Zero Belly Diet*, more and more evidence keeps proving that point. For example, a study in the journal *Evolution and Human Behavior* found that people who ate more portions of red and orange fruits and vegetables had a more sun-kissed complexion than those who ate less—the result of disease-fighting compounds called carotenoids.

ruby red grapefruit, tart cherries, raspberries, strawberries, blueberries, blackberries, red apples (especially Pink Lady), watermelon, plums, peaches, nectarines

OLIVE OIL AND OTHER HEALTHY FATS

Vanquish Hunger

Fat does more than just make our food taste good. In fact, the right kinds of fat, like that found in extra-virgin olive oil, nuts, and avocado, can ward off the munchies by regulating hunger hormones. A study published in *Nutrition Journal* found that participants who ate half a fresh avocado with lunch reported a 40 percent decreased desire to eat for hours afterward. And a brand-new study by scientists in India looked at sixty middle-aged men who were at risk for diabetes and heart disease. They gave the two groups similar diets, except that one of these groups got 20 percent of their daily calories from pistachios. The group that ate the pistachios had smaller waists at the end of the study period!

extra-virgin olive oil, virgin coconut oil, avocados, walnuts, cashews, almonds, almond butter, wild salmon, sardines, ground flaxseed (flax meal), chia seeds

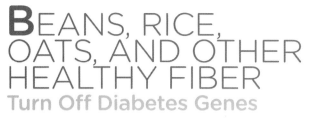

BEANS, RICE, OATS, AND OTHER HEALTHY FIBER
Turn Off Diabetes Genes

Think of beans as little weight-loss pills, and enjoy them whenever you'd like. One study found that people who ate ¾ cup of beans daily weighed 6.6 pounds less than those who didn't, even though the bean eater consumed, on average, 199 more calories per day. Part of the reason is that fiber—from beans and whole grains—helps our bodies produce a substance called butyrate, which deactivates the genes that cause insulin insensitivity.

One common source of fiber that you won't find in these recipes, however, is wheat. Zero Belly isn't strictly a gluten-free program, but all of the recipes in this book use foods that are naturally gluten-free, for a reason: If you have gluten intolerance, then this protein will cause inflammation in your gut. My goal has been to create a plan that will work for everyone. So go ahead and have your Wheaties if you want, but more and more science says that sticking with the Zero Belly fiber sources might make more sense: According to a study in the *Annals of Nutrition and Metabolism*, scientists found that having oatmeal for breakfast resulted in greater fullness, lower hunger ratings, and fewer calories eaten at the next meal compared to a serving of ready-to-eat sugared corn flakes, even though the calorie counts of the two breakfasts were identical.

ZERO BELLY FAVORITES

canned black and garbanzo beans, French green lentils, rolled oats, quinoa, brown rice

EXTRA PROTEIN
Boosts Metabolism

One of the unique qualities of Zero Belly is its reliance on plant-based proteins. While I'm no vegetarian—not by a long shot!—I also know that relying on dairy-based supplements to boost your protein intake isn't always the best bet for those of us focused on gut health—especially those who suffer from lactose intolerance.

ZERO BELLY FAVORITES

Vega One All-in-One Nutritional Shake, Vega Sport Performance Protein, Sunwarrior Warrior Blend, PlantFusion Protein

LEAFY GREENS, GREEN TEA, AND BRIGHT VEGETABLES
Stop Inflammation and Turn Off Fat-Storage Genes

A leafy green like Swiss chard is a veritable Swiss Army knife for weight loss. When you eat more greens, you arm your body with high levels of folate, a B vitamin that's been linked to everything from boosting mood to battling cancer. It's also a key that locks down genes linked to insulin resistance and fat-cell formation.

But leafy greens also perform another important function: They help provide you with a healthy, balanced gut. See, it's not enough to just get beneficial bacteria into your body. To make sure the good guys stay healthy and thrive, you need to feed them. And what they really love is something called fructooligosaccharides, or FOS, a type of fiber found in vegetables as well as fruits and grains. But veggies, because of their low caloric load, are probably the healthiest way of all to get these essential nutrients into your belly. FOS has been shown to increase absorption of vitamins and minerals, improve feelings of fullness, and otherwise keep everything running "clean."

ZERO BELLY FAVORITES

kale, spinach, watercress, romaine, carrots, Swiss chard, zucchini, red bell peppers, tomatoes, cucumbers, celery, asparagus

ZERO BELLY **FOODS**

LEAN MEATS AND FISH
Build Muscle and Turn Off Fat-Storage Genes

Maintaining and building muscle is important, especially as we get older. Increased muscle mass means a healthier weight, better fitness, and improved quality of life. But in order to get those benefits, we may need to eat more protein than we currently do. A lot of this can come from plant proteins in our Zero Belly Drinks. But an extra helping of lean meat might not hurt, either.

Current US recommendations for daily dietary protein are about 0.8 grams per kilogram of body weight, or roughly 62 grams a day for a 170-pound person. A small chicken breast has about 20 grams of protein; so does a serving of ground beef, salmon, or tofu that's about the size of a deck of playing cards. But in a 2015 study in the *American Journal of Physiology—Endocrinology and Metabolism*, researchers found that those who ate twice as much protein as the RDA (Recommended Dietary Allowance) had greater net protein balance and muscle protein synthesis—in other words, it was easier for them to maintain and build muscle.

ZERO BELLY FAVORITES

chicken, lean ground turkey, lean beef, wild salmon, shrimp, scallops, cod, tuna, halibut

ZERO BELLY FOODS

YOUR FAVORITE SPICES

Turn Off Genes for Inflammation and Weight Gain

At my old restaurant White Street, what I got the most compliments on wasn't the exotic cocktails, the beefy steaks, or the rich, creamy desserts. It was the little things like vegetable side dishes, soups, and simple meat dishes such as roast chicken. And that's because the chefs were masters at the art of mixing and maximizing spices. They can make something you've eaten ten thousand times taste like something you've never experienced before.

But herbs, spices, and flavorings do more than add extra pizzazz to your food. From fighting cancer to managing insulin response to fighting inflammation, many popular spices are nutritional stars, and the more you can incorporate them into your daily meals, the better your health and the happier your taste buds.

While most herbs and spices have powerful anti-inflammatory properties, there's a difference between what's in the herb itself and what actually makes its way into your system—what's known as "bioavailability."

To test the actual potency of spices after they've been

ingested, researchers at the University of Gainesville, Florida, and at Penn State had subjects eat significant amounts of different spices every day for a week. Then they tested the subjects' blood plasma by dripping it onto inflamed white blood cells. The plasma of subjects who ate cloves, ginger, rosemary, and turmeric were the most potent—in other words, these spices have the highest level of anti-inflammatory impact after ingestion.

ZERO BELLY FAVORITES

black pepper, turmeric, cinnamon, unsweetened cocoa powder (non-alkalized), cayenne, dried thyme, dried rosemary, dried oregano

SECRET WEAPON

TURMERIC

The super spice has been used for centuries in Indian and Chinese medicine—and for good reason. It contains curcumin, which shrinks your waist, fights chronic inflammation, fights cancer, and boosts levels of BDNF, a brain hormone that promotes neuron growth. It can even treat depression, making for a very good morning.

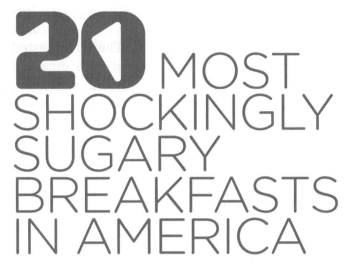

20 MOST SHOCKINGLY SUGARY BREAKFASTS IN AMERICA

"I just can't seem to lose weight," my friend Cassie told me one morning over breakfast. She was drinking a Frappuccino and eating a bowl of granola, rushing to get to work after pressing the snooze button three times.

"Here's your problem," I said, "and your solution: Swap that frap for green tea, replace the granola with eggs, and wake up 10 minutes earlier. Make simple changes like those during every meal and boom: You can lose up to 5 pounds this workweek alone."

"That's a pound a day!" she said.

Exactly.

The American Heart Association recommends no more than 25 grams of added sugar a day for optimal health. Cassie's drink had 65 grams alone. Here are more of the country's worst sugar shockers!

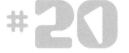

Au Bon Pain Cinnamon Crisp Bagel

370 calories
6 g fat (3 g saturated)
71 g carbs
3 g fiber
25 g sugar
9 g protein

That's more sugar than two glazed Dunkin' Donuts!

With 25 grams of sugar in every Cinnamon Crisp, you'd be better off with a bowl of Cinnamon Toast Crunch, which has one-third the sugar. Worse: If you add cream cheese to the bagel and pair it with a medium Caramel Macchiato, you've just added another 40 grams. Au revoir Au Bon.

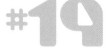

Hardee's Cinnamon 'n' Raisin Biscuit

340 calories
15 g fat (3.5 g saturated)
49 g carbs
1 g fiber
26 g sugar
3 g protein

That's more than two and a half Tootsie Pops' worth of sugar!

When is a biscuit—traditionally a low-sugar food—not a biscuit? When you fill one with raisins and drench them in cinnamon icing. Then it's cake. Order the Smoked Sausage Biscuit instead. You'll save 23 grams of sugar and gain 12 grams of protein. (And P.S. With 21 grams of sugar, Hardee's Blueberry Biscuit isn't much better.)

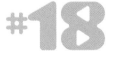

IHOP Chicken & Waffles

1,130 calories
60 g fat (20 g saturated)
108 g carbs
5 g fiber
27 g sugar
41 g protein

That's more sugar than two Baked Apple Pies from McDonald's!

Meet the Jekyll and Hyde of breakfasts: You get protein-packed chicken (healthy enough if you remove the fried skin), paired with dessert-like waffles (run!). And if you add a topping—like IHOP's peach topping—expect another 13 grams of sugar minimum.

Dunkin' Donuts Apple Cheese Danish

400 calories
19 g fat (8 g saturated)
53 g carbs
1 g fiber
29 g sugar
5 g protein

That's the sugar equivalent of two and a half glazed doughnuts from Dunkin'!

Yes, you read that right: This Danish is worth more than doughnuts. Add a medium latte and add another 15 grams of sugar. Instead, skip the danishes all together—none of Dunkin's have fewer than 26 grams of sugar—and get a plain croissant instead. It has only 5 grams of sugar.

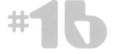

Denny's Steak Skewer & Eggs Skillet

890 calories
50 g fat (14 g saturated)
62 g carbs
4 g fiber
32 g sugar
48 g protein

That's the sugar equivalent of nearly two Snickers bars.

Denny's, home of the Grand Slam, slams you here with hidden sugars. The Steak Skewer & Eggs Skillet consists of a grilled sirloin steak skewer atop fire-roasted bell peppers and onions, mushrooms, and seasoned red-skinned potatoes topped with two eggs. So where's the sugar? It's in the sweet bourbon sauce bathing the steak.

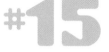

Burger King Ultimate Breakfast Platter

1,190 calories
66 g fat (15 g saturated)
123 g carbs
5 g fiber
32 g sugar
27 g protein

That's the sugar equivalent of 67 M&Ms!

Despite its low price, Burger King's $5 Ultimate Breakfast Platter is the ultimate in getting less for less. The platter features eggs, sausage, hash browns, a biscuit, and three pancakes drizzled in syrup—totaling 32 grams of sugar, with 1,200 calories. Buy a breakfast sandwich instead. The CROISSAN'WICH Egg & Cheese has just 4 grams of sugar and is cheaper, too.

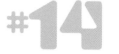

McDonald's Fruit & Maple Oatmeal

310 calories
4 g fat (1.5 g saturated)
62 g carbs
5 g fiber
33 g sugar
6 g protein

That's nearly three doughnuts' worth of sugar!

Plain oatmeal is a Zero Belly Diet staple—its resistant starch will leave you fuller, longer. But McDonald's recipe includes brown sugar and cream in the oatmeal itself and is then topped with diced apples, dried cranberries, and raisins. Similar breakfasts from Denny's and White Castle had 27 grams and 21 grams of sugar, respectively—when ordering oatmeal, make sure it's as plain as possible. Add fresh fruit on top if desired.

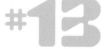

Dunkin' Donuts Blueberry Butternut Donut

490 calories
25 g fat (10 g saturated)
62 g carbs
1 g fiber
37 g sugar
5 g protein

That's nearly as much sugar as a can of Pepsi!!

Not all doughnuts are do-nots. A simple glazed doughnut has only 12 grams of sugar. But you'll triple that when ordering the Blueberry Butternut. To run (faster) on Dunkin', order the bacon, egg, and cheese breakfast sandwich on a croissant instead—more protein, less sugar.

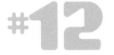

#12

Perkins Belgian Waffle with 2 oz Syrup

610 calories
23 g fat (11 g saturated)
92 g carbs
2 g fiber
39 g sugar
9 g protein

That's as much sugar as you'll find in 10 Pecan Sandies!

Talk about a sticky situation. The Perkins waffle itself—even with a topping of powdered sugar and whipped butter—has only 10 grams of sugar, but when you add just 2 oz of Perkins syrup, that figure jumps to 39 grams. Adding fresh fruit instead would lower the count—and add belly-filling fiber.

#11

Potbelly Yogurt Parfait

434 calories
13 g fat (1 g saturated)
70 g carbs
4 g fiber
51 g sugar
12 g protein

There's more sugar in this yogurt parfait than in four McDonald's Baked Apple Pies!

Yogurt parfaits could rightly be called par-fats, with added sugar hiding in the fruit, granola, honey, and, in some cases, the yogurt itself—but Potbelly's parfait takes the cake with 51 grams of sweet stuff. It stands out on a breakfast menu that's otherwise very low in sugar. Speaking of yogurt parfaits, stay away from the Starbucks and McDonald's versions of this popular breakfast item as well. They have 29 grams and 23 grams of sugar, respectively.

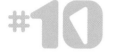

Dunkin' Donuts Coffee Cake Muffin

590 calories
24 g fat (8 g saturated)
87 g carbs
2 g fiber
51 g sugar
7 g protein

That's the sugar equivalent of 65 Jelly Belly jelly beans!

You thought you were making the healthy choice by opting for the muffin instead of the doughnut at Dunkin', but you could have had five Apple 'n' Spice Donuts and still not eaten as much sugar. Add a small latte with almond milk and you're up to 64 g of sugar to start your morning—and crash your afternoon.

The Original Pancake House Apple Waffle

590 calories
31 g fat (18 g saturated)
77 g carbs
1 g fiber
53 g sugar
4 g protein

That's enough sugar for nearly three Snickers bars!

Another waffle derailed by overly sweet toppings. To make matters worse, it's served with whipped butter and hot homemade apple syrup!

IHOP Stuffed French Toast

880 calories
38 g fat (18 g saturated)
119 g carbs
4 g fiber
54 g sugar
15 g protein

That's four and a half doughnuts' worth of sugar on one plate!

What's worse than French toast? Stuffed French toast. This particular variety consists of cinnamon raisin toast stuffed with sweet cream filling, then topped with your choice of strawberry vanilla, peach vanilla, or glazed strawberries. Each order then comes with a dusting of powdered sugar and cool and creamy whipped topping. This is dessert for breakfast.

IHOP Banana Crepes with Nutella

900 calories
45 g fat (13 g saturated)
109 g carbs
6 g fiber
59 g sugar
19 g protein

That's like pouring a 20-ounce Coke on your breakfast!

It's called International House of Pancakes, and IHOP's crepes could cause an international incident. These four are topped with Nutella and equal more than two days' worth of sugar—and that's without any add-ons. Add glazed strawberries and you're adding another 8 grams of sugar.

Sonic Cinnasnacks (5 pc.) with Cream Cheese Frosting

850 calories
43 g fat (17 g saturated)
104 g carbs
7 g fiber
63 g sugar
12 g protein

These cinnasticks have more than five doughnuts' worth of sugar!

Sonic's Cinnasnacks are sweet on their own—they have 29 grams of sugar—but dipped in frosting, you gain another 5 grams of sugar. (This on a breakfast menu thankfully otherwise low on sugar.) Order the breakfast burrito with bacon instead and save more than 60 grams of sugar.

Cinnabon Caramel Pecanbon

1,080 calories
51 g fat (20 g saturated)
146 g carbs
3 g fiber
75 g sugar
14 g protein

That's more than two Cokes' worth of sugar in one bun!

Call this one a Sinnerbon: You get all the sugar of a regular Cinnabon (which has 58 grams of sugar) and add caramel and sugared pecans. Add a Ghirardelli hot chocolate for another 34 grams of sugar and you've had almost 4 days' worth of sugar in one serving!

Denny's Salted Caramel & Banana Cream Pancake Breakfast

1,150 calories
40 g fat (14 g saturated)
184 g carbs
8 g fiber
82 g sugar
15 g protein

You'd need to eat more than six McDonald's Baked Apple Pies to match the sugar found in this breakfast!

This breakfast is about as sugary as they come for Denny's, and we didn't even factor in the meat and egg choice that come with this meal when compiling the nutritional information. One order of these caramel and cream soaked pancakes and you've consumed enough sugar to last more than three days.

IHOP Raspberry White Chocolate Chip Pancakes

850 calories
21 g fat (9 g saturated)
149 g carbs
6 g fiber
83 g sugar
18 g protein

That's nearly seven glazed doughnuts!

Many of IHOP's pancakes are loaded with sugar, but none are quite as sweet as the Raspberry White Chocolate Chip flavor. This dish is made up of four buttermilk pancakes filled with sweet white chocolate chips. It's then crowned with lush raspberry topping, a drizzle of cream cheese icing, and whipped cream.

Perkins Blueberry Pancakes with 2 oz Syrup

1,530 calories
52 g fat (14 g saturated)
248 g carbs
2 g fiber
121 g sugar
16 g protein

This is the sugar equivalent of more than 4 Dairy Queen Vanilla Cones!

Okay, you know pancakes with syrup is gonna be sugary. But holy cow, Perkins, how did you manage to pack nearly five days' worth of sugar into one breakfast? It may seem like a magic trick, but the simple swap of ordering the short stack of pancakes with twin-berry syrup will save you 82 grams of sugar.

Cheesecake Factory French Toast Napoleon with Syrup

2,880 calories
190 g fat (95 g saturated)
1,585 mg sodium
160 g carbs
7 g fiber
139 g sugar
29 g protein

That's the sugar equivalent of five slices of cheesecake!

French Toast Napoleon, meet your Waterloo. This one breakfast will feed you nearly three days' worth of sugar, a day and a half's worth of calories, and nearly a week's worth of saturated fat. Oh, and somehow they squeezed a full day of sodium onto the plate as well!

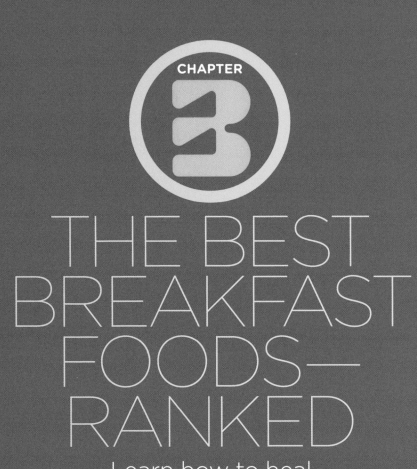

THE BEST BREAKFAST FOODS— RANKED

Learn how to heal
your digestive system with
one simple sip.

S lim people eat breakfast.

That's an indisputable fact, according to a new study from Cornell University. When researchers surveyed 147 slender people who said they'd never had to struggle with their weight, they found that a whopping 96 percent of them ate breakfast nearly every day. (Among the general population, about 28 percent of men and 18 percent of women ages 18 to 34 skip breakfast every day, according to a study by the NPD Group.)

But it's not just eating breakfast that makes slender people seem "naturally skinny." People who manage their weight well tend to eat similar things for breakfast. Fifty-one percent of the slim people surveyed said that on a typical day, their breakfast included a serving of fruit. Forty-one percent said they ate dairy; other popular choices were cold cereal (33 percent), bread (32 percent), eggs (31 percent), and hot cereal (29 percent). And, in one very interesting finding, only 26 percent of slim people said they started their day with coffee.

To help you start blasting belly fat first thing in the morning, me and my friends at Eat This, Not That! dove into the research and uncovered these best-ever weight-loss breakfast foods.

BEST ZERO BELLY BREAKFAST PROTEINS

We've ranked these muscle-building foods from those with the least to the most protein—they're all terrific, but #1 will help tone your arms, legs, chest, and butt fast.

9
Black Beans

Protein, per ½ cup: 7 g

Packed with soluble fiber—a powerful belly fat fighter—beans will not only fill you up for hours but also help slim you down. Wake Forest Baptist Medical Center researchers found that for every 10-gram increase in soluble fiber consumed daily, study participants' belly fat reduced by 3.7 percent over five years. To eat the magical fruit for breakfast, make a Southwestern-inspired omelet filled with black beans, salsa (we like Newman's Own Mild), and nondairy cheese.

8
All Natural Peanut Butter

Protein, per 2 tablespoons: 7-8 g

While processed peanut butter is filled with sugar and waist-widening oils, the real stuff is made with just two ingredients: peanuts and salt. This legume is filled with heart-healthy monounsaturated fats and genistein, a compound that down-regulates fat genes. Nutritionist and personal trainer Kristin Reisinger suggests using the healthy fat in an a.m. smoothie. Take 1 cup of unsweetened almond milk and blend it with 1 scoop of your favorite protein powder, ½ banana, and 1 tablespoon of peanut butter. "This drink is a simple way to start the day with a perfect balance of healthy fats, protein, and carbohydrates to replenish glycogen stores and promote muscle growth, without an overabundance of calories for those seeking weight loss," says Reisinger.

7
Almond Butter
Protein, per 2 tablespoons: 7–8 g
"Almond butter is high in protein, fiber, antioxidants, and monounsaturated fats," says Martha McKittrick, RD, CDN, CDE. "Studies have also shown that people who eat nuts are less likely to become overweight than those who avoid them, likely because it helps you feel fuller, longer." To reap the benefits at breakfast, McKittrick suggests spreading some nut butter on whole-grain toast or adding a tablespoon to oatmeal or smoothies.

6
Eggs
Protein, per two large eggs: 13 g
"Eggs are an excellent source of protein and other healthy nutrients including fat-burning choline," says McKittrick. Choline, also found in lean meats, seafood, and collard greens, attacks the gene mechanism that triggers your body to store fat around your liver, according to *Zero Belly Cookbook*. One test panelist, Morgan Minor, made its egg hash her go-to breakfast, and after just 3 weeks on the program,

the female firefighter lost 11 pounds and 4 inches from her waist! The more eggs you eat, the less egg-shaped you get.

5
Wild Salmon
Protein, per 3 oz: 17 g

"The healthy dose of protein and omega-3 healthy fats found in salmon will keep you satisfied and energized all morning long," says Kristen Carlucci Haase, RDN. "I love smoked salmon and smashed avocado on whole-grain toast, or reheating leftovers of grilled salmon and vegetables for a quick, superfoods-packed start to the day." Just make sure you avoid the farmed variety if weight loss is your goal.

4
Nitrite- and Nitrate-Free Canadian Bacon
Protein, 3 strips: 18 g

Many brands of bacon contain sodium nitrate and nitrite to keep the meat free from harmful bacteria. Under certain conditions, sodium nitrite and nitrate react with amino acids to form cancer-causing chemicals called nitrosamines. And sodium nitrate has been shown to interfere with the body's natural ability to process sugar. However, if you stick with the right variety, bacon can be a healthy, slimming part of your morning meal. Go with Canadian.

3
Chicken Breast
Protein, per 4 oz: 19 g

Chicken may not be your average breakfast food, but maybe it should be. "Some mornings, yogurt or eggs just won't cut it," says Lisa Moskovitz, RD, CDN, CPT, founder of the New York Nutrition Group. "To spice up my breakfast, I'll pull out some leftover dinner, which often contains plenty of fiber-rich veggies and hunger-slashing lean protein. This perfect combination of nutrients keeps me full and energized for hours," she says.

2
Ground Turkey
Protein, per 4 oz: 22 g
If you want to amp up your morning dose of protein, consider adding ground turkey (along with some onions, bell peppers, and mushrooms) to your eggs. The combination is quite tasty and somewhat unexpected, making it a perfect choice for fatigued taste buds. Bonus: The meat is a primo source of DHA omega-3 fatty acids, which have been shown to improve brain function and mood and prevent fat cells from growing.

AND THE #1 BEST PROTEIN FOR BREAKFAST IS...
Organic Protein Powder
Protein, 2 scoops: 34–48 g
Protein powder is the most versatile and nutrient-dense source of the muscle-builder nutrient, earning it a top spot on our list. Use it to make a Zero Belly Smoothie, add it to oatmeal to amp up the protein count, use it to make a homemade nutrition bar, mix it into pancake mix—the options are truly endless.

BEST ZERO BELLY BREAKFAST FRUITS AND VEGGIES

To rank each fruit and veggie, we looked at their fiber and sugar counts, granting points to produce packed with fiber and deducting points from those with more sugar than fiber.

12
Apples

Sugar, per medium fruit: 19 g
Fiber, per medium fruit: 4.4 g

Apples are one of the very best fruit sources of fiber, which, as we said about black beans, is key to blasting belly fat. Throw an apple in your bag along with a nutrition bar and a low-sugar yogurt for a simple, nutrient-filled breakfast on the go.

11
Bananas

Sugar, per fruit: 14 g
Fiber, per fruit: 3 g

"Not only are bananas superstars when it comes to potassium, but they also provide filling fiber and water," says Elisa Zied,

MS, RDN, CDN. She suggests tossing slices of the yellow fruit into unsweetened oatmeal. Smearing slices with some nut butter is another fat-fighting combination worth trying.

10
Grapefruit

Sugar, per ½ cup: 8 g
Fiber, per ½ cup: 1 g

Think of grapefruit (one of the best fruits for fat loss) as your breakfast appetizer. "Even if you changed nothing else about your diet, eating half a grapefruit before each meal may help you lose up to a pound a week," says Patricia Bannan, MS, RDN. "Researchers found that when obese people ate half a grapefruit before each meal, they dropped an average of 3.5 pounds over 12 weeks," she says. How's it work? The tangy fruit helps lower insulin, a fat-storage hormone. It's also 90 percent water, so it fills you up so you eat less, explains Bannan.

9
Berries

Sugar, per ½ cup: 3-7 g
Fiber, per ½ cup: 2-4 g

Berries are one the best fruits for breakfast, hands down. Not only are they "rich in heart-healthy antioxidants, they also provide a generous amount of satiating fiber and vitamins C and K," says Torey Armul, a registered dietitian and spokesperson for the Academy of Nutrition and Dietetics. Berries are also packed with polyphenols, naturally occurring chemicals that aid weight loss and stop fat from forming. Add them to cereal, oatmeal, weight-loss smoothies and shakes, mash them onto peanut butter toast, or nosh on them plain.

8
Tart Cherries
Sugar, per ¹/₂ cup: 6.5 g
Fiber, per ¹/₂ cup: 1.25 g
Tart cherries have been shown to benefit heart health as well as body weight, in a study on obese rats. A 12-week study by the University of Michigan found that rats fed antioxidant-rich tart cherries showed a 9 percent belly fat reduction over rats fed a "Western diet." Moreover, the researchers noted that the cherry consumption had the profound ability to alter the expression of fat genes.

7
Sweet Potatoes
Sugar, per ¹/₂ cup: 7 g
Fiber, per ¹/₂ cup: 2 g
The vibrant tubers are called superfoods for good reason: They're packed with nutrients and can help you burn fat. Sweet potatoes are high in fiber and have a low glycemic index, which means they're absorbed slowly and keep you feeling full longer. Minchen likes to use them to whip up a sweet potato hash. "I love any variation of this dish because it provides rich vitamins, minerals, and fiber from all the veggies. It is very filling, which helps keep appetite and portions under control as the day goes on," she says.

6
Bell Peppers
Sugar, per ¹/₂ cup: 1 g
Fiber, per ¹/₂ cup: 0.8 g
Green, red, or yellow, fresh or frozen, peppers are never a bad companion for your eggs. Thanks to the veggies' high vita-

min C content, eating them can help burn stored fat and convert carbs into fuel. Studies also indicate that vitamin C helps muscles process a fatty acid called carnitine that's essential to muscle growth and recovery. A mere quarter cup of chopped bell peppers—about what you'd add to an omelet—provides 150 percent of the day's recommended intake.

5
Jalapeños

Sugar, per pepper: 0.6 g
Fiber, per pepper: 0.4 g

Registered dietitian Isabel Smith loves spicing up her morning meal—and with good reason: "Thanks to their capsaicin content, spicy peppers can rev the metabolism and may also help to promote satiety, " she explains. "Try adding jalapeño or another spicy pepper to an egg dish or avocado toast," Smith suggests.

4
Broccoli

Sugar, per ½ cup: <1 g
Fiber, per ½ cup: 1 g

Starting the day with cooked or raw veggies is a great way to ensure you get a healthy dose of hard-to-consume nutrients, says Libby Mills, MS, RDN, LDN, FAND "Whether in a smoothie, an omelet, or on an open-faced broiled low-fat cheese sandwich, veggies like broccoli, mushroom, tomato, and onions are loaded with fiber, a nutrient that will help keep you full throughout your busy morning hours," explains Mills.

3
Watermelon

Sugar, per ½ cup: 5 g
Fiber, per ½ cup: 5 g

Watermelon sometimes gets a bad rap for being high in sugar, but the fruit has some impressive health benefits. Research conducted at the University of Kentucky showed that eating watermelon may improve lipid profiles and lower fat accumulation.

2
Spinach

Sugar, per ½ cup: <1 g
Fiber, per ½ cup: 2 g

"Spinach is low in calories but high in fiber, which helps to fill you up," says Armul. It's also a rich source of plant-based omega-3s and folate, which help reduce the risk of heart disease, stroke, and osteoporosis. Use it to amp up the nutrient density of your omelets, smoothies, and egg sandwiches.

AND THE #1 BEST PRODUCE FOR BREAKFAST IS...
Avocados

Sugar, per ¼ fruit: 0.33 g
Fiber, per ¼ fruit: 3.5 g

Avocados—one of the best weight-loss foods on the planet—contain nearly 20 vitamins and minerals in every serving, says McKittrick, including oleic fatty acids, which have been shown to reduce abdominal fat. Avocados are also a good source of fiber and fat. "Use the green fruit to make avocado toast or bake an egg in half of an avocado," McKittrick suggests. See, not all fats are bad.

KITCHEN SECRET

THE CHOCOLATE PUDDING FRUIT!

Known as the "chocolate pudding fruit," black sapote tastes like . . . chocolate pudding. No wonder it's an Eat This, Not That! favorite! Deceptively rich and creamy, a 100-gram serving has 130 calories and 191 mg of vitamin C, or twice that of an orange. (That's a mic-drop chocolate pudding.) A study published in *Food Research International* found black sapote to be a good source of carotenoids and catechins, which spur the release of fat from fat cells and help the liver convert fat into energy.

HOW TO ENJOY IT: Originating in South America, black sapotes can be found in Florida and Hawaii, and certain growers online will ship them within the United States. Devotees swear by them for low-calorie pies and smoothies.

BEST ZERO BELLY BREAKFAST CARBS AND GRAINS

Here, we awarded points for high fiber and protein counts. We then deducted points from products that had a higher sugar count than the competition.

5
Steel-Cut Oatmeal

Fiber per cup: 3 g
Protein per cup: 5 g
Sugar per cup: 6 g

Steel-cut oats are higher in fiber and have a lower glycemic index than other oat varieties, which helps keep bellies full and satisfied hours after eating. While standard steel-cut oats take longer to cook than most other varieties, Pacific Foods offers a pre-cooked, cane sugar–sweetened variety that comes in a convenient grab-and-go box and is ready to eat in just minutes. Just pour it in a bowl, zap it, and eat it as is—there's no need to add water.

4
Crispy Brown Rice

Fiber per cup: 1 g
Protein per cup: 2 g
Sugar per cup: 1 g

Sure they may go "snap, crackle, pop," but these 100 percent whole-grain, gluten-free puffs (I like the Erewhon brand) are a more nutritious choice than the brand you're likely thinking of. This low-sugar cereal carries a slightly nutty flavor and pairs well with both strawberries and raspberries. These fruits provide the hunger-busting fiber this otherwise nutritious cereal lacks, ensuring you'll stay satiated until lunch.

3
Quinoa

Protein per cup, cooked: 8 g
Fiber per cup, cooked: 5.2 g
Fat per cup, cooked: 3.5 g

Though this trendy ancient grain isn't traditionally thought of as a breakfast food, eating it in the a.m. can help start your day off right. You can add the cooked grain to an omelet along with tomatoes, spinach, onions (a veggie that torches stored fat), and a sprinkle of cumin. Alternatively, use quinoa to make overnight oats. Here's Reisinger's go-to recipe: Combine 1 cup of cooked quinoa, ½ cup of unsweetened almond milk, ¼ cup of nonfat Greek yogurt, 1 tablespoon of chia seeds, and 1 teaspoon of vanilla extract. Refrigerate overnight in a Mason jar or covered bowl. In the morning top with ½ cup of berries or half of a sliced banana. "This is a terrific low-sugar way to start the day for those looking to drop a few pounds," Reisinger says.

2
Sprouted-Grain Toast

Protein, 2 slices: 8 g
Fiber, 2 slices: 6 g
Fat, 2 slices: 1 g

Not all breads are carb bombs waiting to shatter your weight-loss goals, and sprouted-grain toast is the very best example of that. This nutrient-dense bread is loaded with folate-filled lentils, protein, and good-for-you grains and seeds such as barley and millet. To boost the flavor of her slices, Marisa Moore, RD, likes to top hers with smashed avocado and smoked salmon—two other foods that made this best breakfast food list! "The healthy fats in the avocado and salmon nourish the heart while the fiber and protein help keep hunger at bay," explains Moore.

AND THE #1 BREAKFAST CARB AND GRAIN IS...
Plain Oatmeal

Fiber per cup, cooked: 4 g
Protein per cup, cooked: 6 g
Sugar per cup, cooked: 1.1 g

"Oatmeal—great source of complex carbohydrates to fuel the body and fiber to decrease the risk of heart disease," says nutrition and fitness expert Jim White, RDN. He suggests pairing oatmeal with blueberries, walnuts, and almond milk for a filling, nutrient-rich morning meal.

BEST ZERO BELLY BREAKFAST TOPPINGS AND MIX-INS

Unlike the other categories on this list, we've ranked the things here by their versatility and overall nutrition and health benefits. Foods that had multiple uses earned extra points, as did things that have been shown to supercharge weight-loss efforts.

7
Black Pepper

Piperine, the powerful compound that gives black pepper its characteristic heat and taste, has been used for centuries in Eastern medicine to treat multiple health conditions including inflammation and tummy troubles. And recent animal studies have found that the compound may also have the ability to block the formation of new fat cells—a reaction known as adipogenesis, resulting in a decrease in waist size, body fat, and cholesterol levels. Season your omelets, breakfast sandwiches, and avocado toast with a few grinds; your waist will thank you.

Walnuts

Richer in heart-healthy omega-3s than salmon, loaded with more anti-inflammatory polyphenols than red wine, and packing half as much muscle-building protein as chicken, the walnut sounds like a Frankenfood, but it grows on trees. Other nuts combine only one or two of these features, not all three. Zied likes to add them to cold cereal bowls, oatmeal, and yogurt. "A small amount provides lots of flavor and texture to meals," notes Zied. A one-ounce serving (which is about seven nuts) is all you need.

5
Ginger

"Ginger contains anti-inflammatory properties and, for some, may help to promote weight loss and overall health," notes Smith. She suggests combining an inch of ginger with carrots and apples to make a refreshing fresh breakfast juice. If juicing isn't your thing, add ginger root to smoothie, pancake, muffin, or oatmeal recipes.

4
Cinnamon

Not only does it taste great, but studies show that cinnamon may help ward off the accumulation of belly fat. "Research also shows that this comforting spice can help with high blood sugars and blood pressure," adds Moskovitz. She suggests adding it to oats, yogurt, or hot coffee. It also fares well in smoothies and homemade pancakes.

3
Flaxseeds

A mere tablespoon of these ultra-powerful seeds serves up nearly 3 grams of belly-filling fiber for just 55 calories. Not to mention, flaxseeds are the richest plant source of omega-3 fats, which help reduce inflammation, ward off mood swings, and help prevent heart disease and diabetes. They make a welcome crunchy addition to smoothies, yogurt, oatmeal, or toast topped with avocado or nut butter, says McKittrick.

2
Chia Seeds

"Chia seeds contain soluble fiber that forms a gel in the stomach," says Smith. This gel slows digestion and promotes satiety, which can help dieters decrease their overall calorie consumption, she explains. Add chia seeds to your a.m. oatmeal, yogurt, or smoothie.

AND THE #1 BREAKFAST MIX-IN IS . . .
Coconut Oil

What smells like an exotic vacation and can shrink your waist faster than almost any other food? Coconut oil! The tropical fat is filled with the medium-chain saturated fat lauric acid, which converts into energy more easily than other types of fat, ultimately aiding weight loss. Don't believe it? Consider this: A study of 30 men in the journal *Pharmacology* found that just 2 tablespoons per day reduced waist circumference by an average of 1.1 inches over the course of a month. Smith suggests using it to grease your egg's frying pan or adding a teaspoon or two into a smoothie.

BEST ZERO BELLY BREAKFAST DRINKS

Imagine going an entire workday without drinking a thing. That's what's happening after a good night's sleep—you wake up dehydrated, making what you drink the first most important decision of the day. Here are our top four picks for what to imbibe.

4

Coffee

One reason slim people stay slender is that they avoid the "Frappuccino"—which is an exotic way of saying you're drinking two ice-cream cones' worth of calories while catching a caffeine buzz. If you absolutely must have your morning buzz, perk yourself up with a nonfat, unsweetened iced coffee instead. And if your sweet tooth must be satisfied, ask your barista to add in two pumps of your favorite flavored syrup to your cup instead of the Frap's four (we like caramel). This simple swap will save you more than 400 calories and a whopping 53 grams of the sweet stuff—that's more sugar than you'll find in three Starbucks chocolate croissants.

3
Spa Water

It's no secret that chugging plain H_2O can be less than stimulating, but there are fun ways to make this healthy habit less of a chore. Certain fruits—such as grapefruit, lemon, and cucumber—have detoxifying properties in their flesh and peels; slice them whole into your water to reap the benefits and hit your water intake quota with an infusion of flavor.

2
Green Tea

We've discovered the most effective weight-loss tool in the world—a weapon that works for everyone, costs just pennies a day, is available at any grocery store, requires no sweat or stress, and can be done at home, at work, or anywhere it's convenient. Literally hundreds of studies have been carried out to document the health benefits of catechins, the group of antioxidants concentrated in the leaves of tea plants. And the most powerful of all catechins, a compound called epigallocatechin gallate, or EGCG, is found almost exclusively in green tea.

AND THE #1 BREAKFAST DRINK IS . . .
Zero Belly Smoothies

Trim people love their protein shakes—and it's easy to see why: Thanks to their high protein content, they aid weight maintenance by boosting calorie burn and satiety and preserving lean muscle mass. But when getting a flat belly is your goal, choosing the right protein powder is key. Because whey is a dairy derivative—and commercial preparations tend to contain all manner of funky chemicals—protein powders that use this source as a base can lead to bloat. Plant protein powders, such as those used in Zero Belly Smoothies, won't.

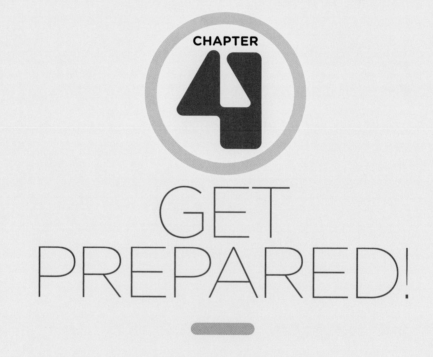

CHAPTER

4

GET
PREPARED!

I f you own a pan, a carton of eggs, and a bottle of extra-virgin olive oil, you've already got the tools to make a healthy breakfast. Here we give you the tools to make a Zero Belly Breakfast—one that's delicious and high in protein, and effortlessly melts fat.

It's a culmination of two decades in the kitchen, developing recipes for Eat This, Not That!, it's sister series Cook This, Not That!, and the Zero Belly franchise. And the best part is, these picks won't only save you calories—they'll save you money, too. A lot of it.

Cooking at home has been irrefutably proven to do so. "Depending on how frequently you eat out," estimates nutritionist Lauren Minchen, "cooking your food at home can save you hundreds of dollars a month."

A 2017 federal data study backs her up, showing that grocery expenses are 2 percent lower than last year, "the first decline in prices since 1967," owing to lower transportation costs, a strong US dollar, and increased production. Meanwhile, the average cost for food eaten out rose 2.6 percent—in fact, spending on restaurants and bars surpassed groceries for the first time ever!

Save a calorie, save a dollar. The brands mentioned are some of our favorites, and, speaking of money, we were not paid to mention them. If you prefer other brands, be our guest. We just ask that we be *your* guest next time you're whipping up the Mile-High Omelet.

Choose your protein powder

The sheer number of protein supplements on store shelves will make your head spin like the blades of a blender. Simplify your world by understanding that there are two main categories: animal-based protein supplements made from eggs, whey, and casein, and plant-based forms from pea, hemp, rice, and soy proteins. Zero Belly advocates solely plant-based protein powders because studies show that vegetable proteins may have a more powerful weight-loss effect than animal proteins. And because they're lactose-free and usually lower in sugar, vegan proteins do a better job of fighting bloat and inflammation. (Just avoid soy.)

Any good protein powder will provide at least 15 grams of protein per serving. Choosing a blended plant-protein powder (containing pea, rice, and a variety of sprouts, for example) will ensure you're getting more amino acids. You'll want to have a tub handy for Zero Belly Smoothies, but also to mix into cereals, add to pancakes, or sprinkle onto a warm waffle. Here are our go-to favorites.

KASHI GOLEAN PLANT POWERED SHAKE

Made of greens, beets, and sprouted legumes, this is the most easily mixable plant protein powder we've tried—and one of the most delicious, coming in flavors like Dark Cocoa Power and Vanilla Vinyasa.

2 scoops
180 calories
7 g fat (1 g saturated fat)
13 g carbs
1 g sugar
21 g protein

VEGA ONE ALL-IN-ONE NUTRITIONAL SHAKE

A blend of vegan proteins, Vega gives you everything you need in one dose. Vega Sport Performance Protein will do the same.

1 scoop
170 calories
6 g fat (0 g trans fat)
13 g carbs
>1 g sugar
20 g protein

SUNWARRIOR WARRIOR BLEND RAW VEGAN PROTEIN

With 19 grams of protein and 100 calories per serving, this organic protein is derived from peas, cranberries, and hemp, with no sugars, gluten, or artificial sweeteners to cause a metabolism-confusing midday crash. But it's tasty enough to take on its own. If you down some pre-workout, the branched-chain amino acids can give your gym session a boost.

1 scoop
100 calories
2 g fat (0 g saturated fat)
2 g carbs
0 g sugar
19 g protein

GARDEN OF LIFE RAW MEAL

This organic protein blend, good for a meal replacement, is derived from belly-fat-blasting brown rice, quinoa, and beans, plus tea and cinnamon extract. With 34 grams of protein and 10 grams of fiber per two-scoop serving, having one of these for lunch before a workout will keep you feeling full and energized while preserving muscle.

1 scoop
155 calories
2.5 g fat (1 g saturated fat)
16 g carbs
3.5 g sugar
17 g protein

ALIVE! ULTRA-SHAKE PEA PROTEIN

Pea protein is rich in amino acids and is easy to digest. While not as preferable as a full blend, this variety by Alive! contains a substantial 15 grams of protein per scoop, plus a multivitamin's worth of nutrients.

1 scoop
120 calories
>1 g fat (0 g saturated fat)
15 g carbs
9 g sugar
15 g protein

NUTIVA ORGANIC HEMP PROTEIN

Stifle the Woody Harrelson jokes: Hemp protein is derived from the less-fun parts of the hemp plant, offering a substantial amount of fiber (here, 8 grams) that's easy to digest.

With 15 grams of protein per scoop, this organic option is an ideal mix-in for oatmeal or smoothies (or brownies, if that's your thing); the fiber will make you feel fuller longer, and it contains eight essential amino acids to build muscle.

1 scoop
90 calories
3 g fat (0 g saturated fat)
9 g carbs
1 g sugar
15 g protein

Choose your milk

Fans of Zero Belly Smoothies know how fun it is to mix and match plant-based milks—almond and coconut are the most prevalent, but don't be afraid to substitute hemp, rice, oat, or hazelnut varieties, as long as all are unsweetened. One to skip: soy milk. Highly concentrated doses of soy can have a negative impact on lean muscle tissue, thanks to the estrogen-like chemicals that occur naturally in the plant.

Outfit your kitchen

Saunter down to Williams-Sonoma and pick up a 15-piece All-Clad stainless steel cookware set and you'll drop $2,000. Tack on a set of Henckels knives, a 15-piece tool set, and a few gadgets and you're out over $2,600 before you've made your first omelet. Truth is, you need only a few all-purpose pots, pans, and tools to turn out four-star food from your kitchen every morning (and night), and quality and price don't always correlate in the kitchen. We've highlighted the essentials and our favorite affordable picks in each category. All told, we'll have your kitchen fully outfitted for less than the cost of a fancy breakfast meeting at the Ritz.

Nonstick Skillets

CALPHALON CONTEMPORARY NONSTICK 10" AND 12" OMELETTE PANS ($60+)

In his memoir, *Kitchen Confidential*, Anthony Bourdain detailed the most important test of all when choosing a good pan: Imagine cracking someone's head with the pan, he says. "If you have any doubts about which will dent—the victim's head or your pan—then throw that pan right in the trash." Not only would these skillets crack a hard skull, the slick, durable nonstick coating will last for years.

Best for: Scrambles, omelets, sautéed vegetables, and fish

Cast-Iron Skillet

LODGE LOGIC 12" SKILLET ($34)

It's what our moms used, and our moms' moms, and their moms' moms. . . . After all these years, a better cooking implement simply does not exist. Cast iron holds heat extremely well, making it perfect for developing the type of crust on a thick steak or burger that only a grill could match. A seasoned skillet develops a natural nonstick layer, making it adept at more delicate tasks, too, like frying eggs, cooking fish, and sautéing vegetables. Lodge has been in the cast-iron game since 1896 and still makes one of the finest skillets you'll ever lay a spatula on.

Best for: Seared steak, burgers, blackened fish, pan-frying

Medium Saucepan

CALPHALON CONTEMPORARY NONSTICK 2½-QUART SHALLOW SAUCEPAN WITH LID ($65)

Fancy stainless steel and copper sauciers are worth the money if you spend 8 hours a day in the kitchen. For the rest of us, this sturdy saucepan holds and distributes heat well enough for delicate and aggressive tasks alike.

Best for: Simmering sauces, cooking grains, reheating leftovers

Cutting Board

OXO GOOD GRIPS 21″ X 14½″ ($25)

If you have the cash, go ahead and buy a thick, heavyset wooden cutting board for most of your major chopping, slicing, and dicing. But if you want an affordable, all-purpose board, this is it. The polypropylene material is nonporous (preventing bacteria buildup) and won't dull your knives.

Best for: Tackling a few jobs at once—the surface area is large enough. Save one side for produce and herbs and the other for raw meat.

Chef's Knife

VICTORINOX FORSCHNER FIBROX 8″ ($46)

While the market for handforged $300 Japanese and German chef's knives continues to spiral out of control, the best knife out there may just be this humble blade. Made by the same fine people who brought you the Swiss Army knife, this one blade can handle 90 percent of your cutting. *Cook's Illustrated*, the master of in-depth product tests, has awarded this knife their top seal of approval year after year.

Best for: Most big cutting jobs, including chopping vegetables, meat, and herbs

Serrated Knife

VICTORINOX FORSCHNER FIBROX 10¼″ BREAD KNIFE ($50)

It's always good to have one blade on hand that can cut through everything. This is that blade.

Best for: Slicing bread, tomatoes, citrus fruit, and sandwiches

Pepper Mill

(about $13)

Seems like a small thing, and it is, but great cooking is all about doing the small things well. Shake pepper from a preground container and you've already lost all of its fragrant, fruity spice. If you want one way to improve your food instantly, buy an inexpensive pepper mill, fill it with whole peppercorns, and get your grind on.

Grater

MICROPLANE CLASSIC ZESTER/GRATER ($12)

Never buy cooking tools that do just one job (we're looking

at you, cherry pitter). The Microplane uses hundreds of tiny teeth to make quick work of hard cheese like Parmesan, citrus zest, and whole spices like nutmeg.

Kitchen utensils

Forget the space-wasting, cash-burning 15-piece kitchen tool sets. These are the only three utensils you need.

ONEIDA STAINLESS STEEL LOCKING 9½″ TONGS ($6)

Tongs are the perfect all-purpose kitchen tool, equally adept at turning meat on a grill as they are at plucking pasta strings from boiling water to taste for doneness.

OXO GOOD GRIPS NYLON FLEXIBLE TURNER ($7)

One thing tongs are lousy for: handling delicate foods like fish. For that, Oxo's turners are ideal—especially since they won't scratch your non-stick pans.

OXO GOOD GRIPS LARGE WOODEN SPOON ($6)

Great for stirring sauces, wok maneuvering, whipping milk and butter into mashed potatoes, and sneaking chili tastes when no one is looking.

Blenders

The fact is, you need a quality blender in order to make quality Zero Belly Smoothies. That old model from your dorm room won't be able to crush the ice and frozen fruit quickly enough, which means it can melt and ultimately dilute your precious creation rather than giving it that bracing, velvety texture you want. Here are some of the models we like:

CUISINART POWEREDGE 1,000-WATT BLENDER

An easy-to-use and versatile blender that's great for everything from your fitness-minded smoothies to the kids' strawberry milkshakes.

KITCHENAID 5-SPEED DIAMOND BLENDER

Does it all for a reasonable price.

KITCHENAID 5-SPEED HAND BLENDER

If you travel a lot or like to mix it up in the office, this handy tool is a great solution.

MAGIC BULLET

A small, handheld device that makes blending simple.

NINJA MASTER PREP

A high-speed blender that won't take up a lot of room on your countertop.

NINJA ULTIMA BLENDER 244

This professional-grade blender may be a bit more expensive, but it can muscle its way through just about any food and is easy to clean.

NUTRIBULLET

Perfect for blending while traveling.

VITAMIX 5200

Gorgeous, high-powered, and expensive. But worth it if you blend a lot and want to show off to your nosy friends.

Gadgets

None of these are essential, per se, but they sure are fun.

PADERNO SPIRALIZER

This kitchen gadget-of-the-moment makes spiral cuts, shoestrings, and "noodles" out of your favorite veggies. If you've been jonesing for some pasta since going Paleo or gluten-free, you're going to love all the yummy dishes you can whip up with this. Zucchini and carrot "pasta," anyone? How about some homemade curly sweet potato hash browns?

BLUAPPLE

How many times have you shelled out cash on fresh fruits and veggies, only to find them rotting in your refrigerator before you were able to enjoy them? It's beyond frustrating—and a waste of money, too. The solution: BluApple, a gadget that absorbs the ethylene gas in your fridge that's responsible for rotting your apples and berries (two of our favorite overnight oat toppers).

INSTANT POT

This is the exact opposite of a slow cooker. Instead of waiting 8 hours for your tender beef, you can get it in just 30 minutes, or cook rice in five.

S'WELL BOTTLE

It keeps your spa water cold for 24 hours or your green tea hot for 12—and it's double-walled, stainless steel, and BPA-free.

PEACHY KEEN

Try this deliciously creamy drink in your new blender. It's from *Zero Belly Smoothies*, a perfect companion to *Zero Belly Breakfasts*.

YOU'LL NEED

1 cup frozen peaches

½ banana

1 cup unsweetened almond milk

1 teaspoon vanilla extract

⅓ cup vanilla plant-based protein powder

½ cup ice cubes

Water to blend (optional)

HOW TO MAKE IT

1. Blend all of the ingredients and enjoy!

287 calories
3 g fat (0 g saturated)
5 g fiber
22 g sugar
29 g protein

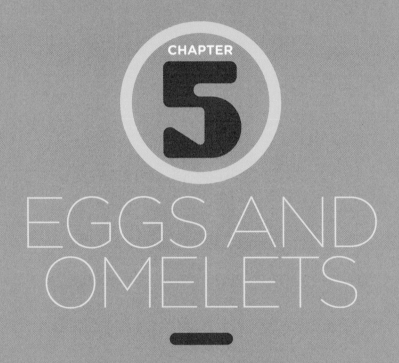

CHAPTER

5

EGGS AND OMELETS

—

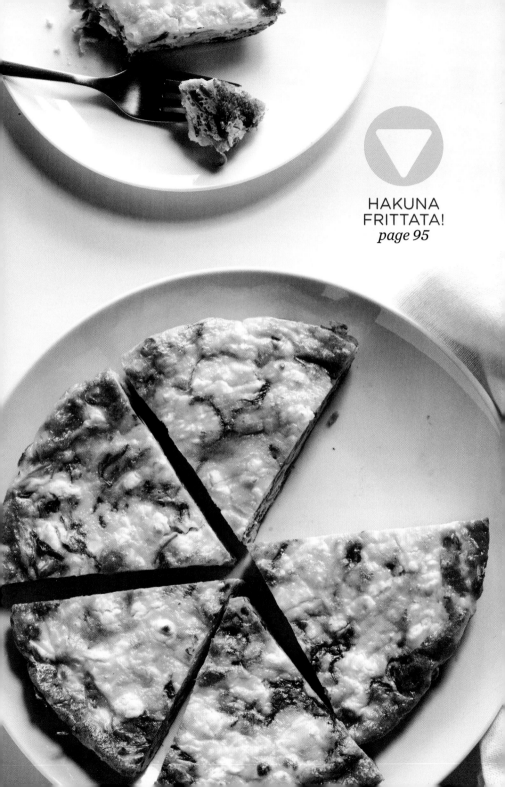

HAKUNA
FRITTATA!
page 95

Tired of scrambling around for breakfast ideas? Feeling fried after a long day's work? Have egg on your face, because you just can't lose that extra three pounds? This chapter's for you.

Eggs are the perfect superfood—high in protein, with zero carbs or fat—and they're the single best dietary source of the B vitamin choline, an essential nutrient used in the construction of all the body's cell membranes. Two eggs will give you half your day's worth; only beef liver has more. (And believe us, starting your day with a slab of beef liver does not make for a great morning.)

Choline deficiency is linked directly to the genes that cause the accumulation of belly fat. Eggs can solve the problem: Research has shown dieters who eat eggs for breakfast as compared to a high-carb meal of a bagel have an easier time losing weight due to their satiety value.

At about 70 calories, a hard-boiled egg also makes an easy afternoon snack . . . just don't tell your coworkers; according to a personality analysis by the British Egg Industry Council, boiled egg consumers tend to be disorganized! (Other findings: fried egg fans have a high sex drive and omelet eaters are self-disciplined.) Discover which kind you are inside. . . .

TACOS LOCOS

Why go to Taco Bell for breakfast when the border's so close to home? This protein-packed taco has sausage and black beans and the healthy fats of an avocado. Kids will love them, too.

YOU'LL NEED

1 egg, lightly beaten

1 link chicken or turkey sausage, chopped

2 tablespoons chopped red onion

1 gluten-free tortilla

¼ cup black beans

2 tablespoons mashed avocado

2 tablespoons salsa

HOW TO MAKE IT

1. Using a nonstick pan, scramble the egg; add the chopped sausage and onion and cook until heated through.

2. Add the egg mixture to the tortilla. Top with beans, avocado, and salsa.

Makes 1 serving
422 calories
16.1 g fat (2.4 g saturated)
556 mg sodium
10.5 g fiber
4.3 g sugar
21.9 g protein

HUEVOS RANCHEROS

Erin Bloys, a chef friend of ours who trained at Le Cordon Bleu, created this for Zero Belly. "We could eat this every day without getting tired of it," she says about her family. We have—and agree.

YOU'LL NEED

4 tablespoon extra-virgin olive oil,

Four 6-inch stone-ground corn tortillas

½ cup Amy's Organic Refried Black Beans

6 ounces baby spinach

⅛ teaspoon cayenne pepper

4 large eggs

1 large avocado, pitted, peeled, chopped

4 tablespoons crumbled queso fresco

1 tablespoon chopped cilantro

Salt and black pepper, to taste

Cholula Original Hot Sauce, to taste

HOW TO MAKE IT

1. In a 12-inch nonstick skillet over medium-high heat, add 1 tablespoon of olive oil. When the oil is hot, quickly sauté two tortillas until crispy on both sides. Repeat with remaining tortillas.

2. Place 2 tortillas on each plate. Spread ⅛ cup of refried black beans over each tortilla.

3. In the same skillet, add another tablespoon of olive oil, the baby spinach, and the cayenne. Sauté until the leaves are wilted. Divide the spinach and top each tortilla with the spinach.

4. Reduce the heat to medium. In the same skillet, add the remaining 2 tablespoons of olive oil. Gently crack the eggs into the pan. Cover with a lid and cook the eggs until the whites are completely set but the yolks are still soft. Using a spatula, place an egg on each tortilla.

5. Top off each plate with half the chopped avocado, 2 tablespoons of queso fresco, ½ tablespoon of cilantro, and salt, pepper, and hot sauce.

Makes 2 servings
411 calories
31.6 g fat (6.5 g saturated)
288 mg sodium
22 g carbs
7.3 g fiber
1.3 g sugar
13.6 g protein

BAKED EGGS
WITH BABY SHIITAKE MUSHROOMS

Packed with protein and healthy fats, this dish will make you feel younger. But it'll make you *look* younger, too. A study in the journal *Biological Trace Element Research* found premature-graying individuals had significantly lower copper levels than a control group. And shiitake mushrooms are one of the best dietary sources of copper. Just a half cup provides 71 percent of your recommended daily intake—and for only 40 calories!

KITCHEN SECRET: Dried shiitake mushrooms have the highest level of fat-blasting choline of any vegetable— one serving has almost double the amount found in an egg yolk.

Makes 1 serving
244 calories
14.1 g fat (3.4 g saturated)
268 mg sodium
16.5 g carbs
1.3 g fiber
2 g sugar
15.3 g protein

YOU'LL NEED

1 teaspoon extra-virgin olive oil

¼ cup chopped red onion

1 cup chopped baby shiitake mushrooms

1 cup spinach

2 eggs

Salt and black pepper, to taste

HOW TO MAKE IT

1. Preheat the oven to 400°F. Grease a 16-oz oven-safe ramekin, using a minimal amount of olive oil.

2. Heat the olive oil in a skillet over medium heat and sauté the onions until soft.

3. Add the mushrooms and spinach; cook until softened.

4. Add the onions, mushrooms, and spinach to the prepared ramekin.

5. Beat the eggs in a small bowl, then pour over onions, mushrooms, and spinach.

6. Bake in the oven for 20 to 25 minutes, or until the egg is set.

7. Salt and pepper to taste.

EGGS IN A HOLE

by Toby Amidor, MS, RD, nutrition expert, and author of *The Greek Yogurt Kitchen*

Our mothers are at war over the proper name of this dish—"framed egg" vs. "toad in the puddle." We'll let you tell them it's actually called "Eggs in a Hole."

YOU'LL NEED

2 plum tomatoes, chopped (about 1 cup)

1 avocado, diced

⅛ teaspoon salt

⅛ teaspoon black pepper

4 slices of 100% whole-wheat bread

2 teaspoons extra-virgin olive oil

Nonstick cooking spray

4 large eggs

HOW TO MAKE IT

1. In a small bowl, combine the tomatoes, avocado, salt, and pepper; set aside.

2. Using a cookie cutter, cut out a hole in the center of each slice of bread. Brush ½ teaspoon olive oil on each slice of bread.

3. Spray a nonstick skillet with nonstick cooking spray and heat over medium-high heat. Place the oiled bread in the pan and gently place a cracked egg in the center hole. Cook until the egg hardens and carefully flip over. Repeat with the remaining bread.

4. Place each egg-filled slice of bread on a plate and top with one-quarter of the tomato-avocado mixture.

Makes 4 servings
Per slice:
278 calories
18.2 g fat
  (4.2 g saturated)
287 mg sodium
19.5 g carbs
6 g fiber
4.7 g sugar
11.6 g protein

Says Toby: "This makes a great breakfast as you're including three food groups in your diet first thing in the morning, and all the good-for-you nutrients that come with them. Whole grains are satisfying and provide fiber and several B-vitamins, eggs are a perfect protein and provide the antioxidant lutein, and the vegetables in the tomato-avocado mixture provide vitamin C and a boatload of unsaturated healthy fat!"

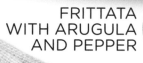

FRITTATA
WITH ARUGULA
AND PEPPER

FRITTATA
WITH ARUGULA AND PEPPER

At its core, a frittata is a crustless quiche that's both considerably easier to make and substantially healthier to eat. Make one at the beginning of the week, then slice off a wedge each morning for breakfast. You could even stuff a piece in a toasted gluten-free English muffin for a gourmet breakfast sandwich.

YOU'LL NEED

½ **tablespoon extra-virgin olive oil**

¼ **cup bottled roasted red peppers,** chopped

1 clove garlic, minced

4 cups baby arugula or baby spinach

4 thin slices prosciutto or other good ham, cut into strips

8 eggs, beaten

Salt and black pepper, to taste

½ **cup crumbled goat cheese**

FRITTATA WITH
ARUGULA AND PEPPER
continuation

HOW TO MAKE IT

1. Preheat the broiler. Heat the olive oil in a nonstick, 12-inch oven-safe skillet over medium-low heat. Add the roasted pepper and garlic and cook for about 1 minute, until the garlic is fragrant but not browned. Stir in the arugula and cook for about 2 minutes more, until lightly wilted. Add the prosciutto, then pour the eggs over the top. Season the eggs with a good amount of salt and pepper, then dot with the crumbled goat cheese.

2. Cook on the stovetop for 5 to 6 minutes, until most of the egg has set. Place the pan 6 inches under the broiler and cook for about 3 minutes, until the rest of the egg has fully set and the top of the frittata has begun to brown. Cool slightly, remove from the pan, and cut into wedges.

Makes 4 servings
233 calories
16 g fat (5.6 g saturated)
488 mg sodium
3.3 g carbs
0.6 g fiber
2.1 g sugar
17.4 g protein

KITCHEN SECRET

HAKUNA FRITTATA!

Don't take the ingredients in this recipe too literally; rather, learn the basic technique, then play around with the filling based on what you like or what your refrigerator happens to be sheltering. Here are a few ideas to get the wheels turning:

• Sautéed chorizo, onions, and poblano peppers

• Leftover chicken or steak, pesto, and ricotta cheese

• Mushrooms, spinach, sun-dried tomatoes, and feta

SWEET POTATO EGG BOATS

One large, flavor-packed spud serves up 4 grams of satiety-boosting protein, 25 percent of the day's belly-filling fiber, and 11 times the recommended daily intake of vitamin A, a nutrient that aids immune function, vision, reproduction, and cellular communication. Sweet!

YOU'LL NEED

1 baked sweet potato

2 eggs

¼ teaspoon cumin

¼ teaspoon turmeric

¼ teaspoon chili powder

Salt and black pepper, to taste

Aquafaba (see recipe on page 188)

1 tablespoon nutritional yeast

HOW TO MAKE IT

1. Preheat the oven to 400°F.

2. Cut the baked sweet potato in half and place it in a baking dish. Scoop out the insides, leaving about ¼ inch cushion. Crack an egg into each half.

3. Mix together the cumin, turmeric, and chili powder and sprinkle over the egg (go lightly if you don't like too much spice, or use it all if you do like spicy). Season with salt and pepper to taste.

4. Bake in the oven for 20 to 25 minutes, or until the egg is set.

5. FOR TOPPING: Mix ½ cup of the frothed aquafaba with nutritional yeast to make a savory creamy topping.

KITCHEN SECRET: Sweet potatoes can be used to make burgers and quinoa cakes, added to mouthwatering salads, or mixed in a breakfast quinoa bowl.

Makes 1 serving
Calculated without aquafaba
270 calories
9.8 g fat (2.8 g saturated)
178 mg sodium
29.9 g carbs
6.8 g fiber
8.2 g sugar
18.2 g protein

PORTOBELLO ROAD
WITH BACON AND JALAPEÑOS

Is it any wonder why ancient Egyptians believed snacking on mushrooms was the key to a long life? Portobellos contain the highest vegetable source of inflammation-fighting vitamin D, and researchers at the University of Florida discovered that people who munched on just four ounces of cooked mushrooms every day for four weeks showed increased immunity.

YOU'LL NEED

Portobello mushroom cap (about 4-inch diameter)

1 tablespoon extra-virgin olive oil

¼ **jalapeño pepper,** chopped (or more if you're brave)

1 slice uncured Canadian bacon, chopped

½ **cup baby spinach**

1 egg

Salt and black pepper, to taste

Parsley, to taste

HOW TO MAKE IT

1. Preheat the oven to 375°F.

2. Prepare the mushroom: Remove the stem and gills. Rub 1 to 2 teaspoons of olive oil all over the mushroom cap and place it upside down into a small baking dish or ramekin.

3. Heat 1 teaspoon oil in a small frying pan. Sauté the jalapeño and Canadian bacon for 2 to 3 minutes or until they begin to brown.

4. Tear the spinach into smaller pieces and put into the mushroom cap. Add the pepper/bacon mixture on top of the spinach. Crack the egg on top of the pepper/bacon. Add salt, pepper, and parsley to taste.

5. Bake until the egg sets.

KITCHEN SECRET: Jalapeños, habaneros, and cayenne peppers all get their fiery bite from a naturally occurring chemical called capsaicin, which boosts metabolism.

Makes 1 serving
210 calories
19 g fat (3.5 g saturated)
247 mg sodium
2 g carbs
0.6 g fiber
1.1 g sugar
10 g protein

PEPPER-UPPERS

You may have heard that spicy hot peppers can help you scorch calories, but did you know that mild peppers can have the same effect? Thanks to a metabolism-boosting compound, dihydrocapsiate, and their high vitamin-C content, red and green bell peppers can help you lose weight.

YOU'LL NEED

1 bell pepper

1 teaspoon extra-virgin olive oil

2 pieces uncured Canadian bacon

½ cup baby spinach, torn up

1 egg

1 teaspoon nutritional yeast

Salt and black pepper

KITCHEN SECRET: Use nutritional yeast to make a vegan mac-and-cheese, sprinkle on your popcorn, or whip up a cheesy soup.

HOW TO MAKE IT

1. Preheat the oven to 375°F.

2. Cut the bell pepper in half, horizontally. Set the bottom half of the pepper in a small baking dish or ramekin and bake in the oven for 10 to 15 minutes.

3. Chop the top half of the bell pepper.

4. Heat the olive oil in small frying pan and sauté the Canadian bacon and the chopped bell pepper until the bacon is slightly browned and the bell pepper is soft.

5. Take the bottom half of the bell pepper out of the oven and line it with the bacon slices. Add the spinach and sautéed bell pepper on top of the bacon. Crack the egg over the spinach and sautéed bell pepper.

6. Bake in the oven for 15 to 20 minutes, or until the egg is set.

7. Top with the nutritional yeast and salt and pepper to taste.

Makes 1 serving
196 calories
10.6 g fat (2.4 g saturated)
425 mg sodium
12.1 g carbs
2.8 g fiber
7.1 g sugar
16 g protein

MEDITERRANEAN HASH

by Libby Mills, MS, RDN, LDN, FAND

Go Greek, with this oil-and-vinegar delight.

YOU'LL NEED

1 teaspoon extra-virgin olive oil

1 clove fresh garlic, minced
    or ⅛ teaspoon garlic powder

½ cup chickpeas, rinsed and drained

¼ cup diced red bell peppers

¼ cup water-packed canned artichokes,
    drained and chopped

1 tablespoon balsamic vinegar

1 cup fresh baby spinach

¼ cup grape tomatoes, halved

1 scallion, chopped

¼ teaspoon fresh dill, chopped
    or ⅛ teaspoon dried dill

Salt and black pepper, to taste

Olive oil spray

1 egg

2 sprigs fresh dill, for garnish

HOW TO MAKE IT

1. Over medium heat, warm a medium sauté pan. Heat the olive oil and add the garlic. Stirring, cook the garlic 30 seconds before mixing in the chickpeas, bell peppers, and artichokes. Cook for 3 to 5 minutes until everything is hot. Incorporate the balsamic vinegar, spinach, tomatoes, scallion, and dill. Lightly season with salt and black pepper as desired. Immediately make a well in the center of the hash. Spray the bottom of the pan with olive oil and add the raw egg, being careful not to break the yolk.

2. Immediately cover and reduce the heat to medium-low. Cook 2 minutes more, allowing the spinach to wilt and the egg to cook. (I cook my egg 3 to 4 minutes because I like my eggs cooked solid.)

3. Serve the hash with the egg on top. Top with a few sprigs of fresh dill.

VARIATION: Add a few crushed red pepper flakes when sautéing the garlic.

Makes 2 servings

265 calories
7.8 g fat (1.4 g saturated)
165 mg sodium
36.3 g carbs
10.8 g fiber
7.9 g sugar
14.2 g protein

Says Libby: "In one pan, all the Mediterranean flavors I love come together in minutes. The sunny-side up presentation of protein on a colorful backdrop of fiber and plenty of vegetables make my Mediterranean Hash the perfect fuel to start my day."

ZERO BELLY EGGS BENEDICT

This is a favorite from *Zero Belly Cookbook*, which has 150+ delicious recipes to flatten your belly and turn off your fat genes, created by master chef Jason Lawless. For a lower-calorie option, substitute four portobello mushroom caps for the English muffins.

YOU'LL NEED

2 gluten-free English muffins, split in half

4 eggs

Olive oil spray

2 cups packed spinach leaves

2 tablespoons mayonnaise

Smoked paprika, to taste (optional)

HOW TO MAKE IT

1. Toast the English muffin halves until golden brown.

2. Poach 4 eggs.

3. While the eggs are poaching, heat a medium sauté pan over medium heat; spray with olive oil spray, and add the spinach. Use a rubber spatula to stir the spinach until wilted. Transfer to a plate lined with paper towels to drain any excess water.

4. Top each toasted English muffin half with one-quarter of the spinach mixture, and 1 poached egg.

5. Top with ½ tablespoon mayonnaise and a pinch of smoked paprika, if desired.

KITCHEN SECRET: Make your own Zero Belly Mayo with 2 egg yolks, the juice of 1 lemon, ½ teaspoon Dijon mustard, ¼ teaspoon kosher salt, and 1 cup extra-virgin olive oil. Pulse the eggs yolks, lemon juice, mustard, and salt in the bowl of a food processor for a second, and then turn it on, pouring in the olive oil until it emulsifies.

Makes 4 servings

177 calories
10.1 g fat (2.4 g saturated)
240 mg sodium
13.5 g carbs
1.3 g fiber
1.4 g sugar
8.5 g protein

THE PERFECT OMELET

Cooking an omelet is like scrambling a batch of eggs, only you let it set in a single unified layer before adding your filling. Follow the steps below.

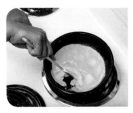 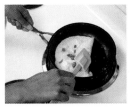 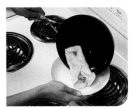

Step 1:
Let the raw egg slide underneath the cooked egg.

Step 2:
When the egg is set, fold the ends over the filling.

Step 3:
Slide the omelet out onto a warm plate.

MILE-HIGH
OMELETS
page 108

MILE-HIGH OMELETS

The classic diner omelet is an oversize envelope of eggs soaked in cheap oil and bulging with fatty fillers. The damage, with toast and hash browns: about 1,400 calories and 70 grams of fat. Our ode to Denver doesn't cut the cheese or the meat or even turn to Egg Beaters. No, this is just honest cooking with good ingredients in reasonable portions, exactly what an omelet should be.

YOU'LL NEED

½ **tablespoon extra-virgin olive oil,**
  plus more for cooking the omelets

1 green bell pepper, diced

4 ounces cremini or button mushrooms, sliced

1 small onion, diced

4 ounces smoked ham,
  cubed or sliced into thin strips

Salt and black pepper, to taste

8 eggs

2 tablespoons almond milk

HOW TO MAKE IT

1. Heat the olive oil in a medium sauté pan over medium heat. Add the bell pepper, mushrooms, and onion and cook for about 7 minutes, until the vegetables are soft and lightly browned. Add the ham, cook for 1 minute more, then season with salt and pepper.

2. Combine the eggs and milk and whisk until fully blended. Season with a few pinches of salt.

3. Heat a small nonstick pan over medium heat. Swirl with just enough olive oil to coat.

4. Ladle in one-quarter of the eggs and as soon as they begin to set, use a wooden spoon to scrape the egg from the bottom, working from one side of the pan to the other (like you were scrambling eggs). Stop scraping just before the egg is fully cooked, then spread one-quarter of the vegetable mixture across the omelet. Use a spatula to carefully fold the egg over on itself.

5. Slide the omelet out onto a warm plate. Repeat to make 4 omelets.

Makes 4 servings
211 calories
13.2 g fat (3.8 g saturated)
502 mg sodium
6.6 g carbs
1.5 g fiber
3.4 g sugar
17.2 g protein

GREEN EGGS & BACON OMELET

Wake up skinnier—and happier. Asparagus is one of the top plant-based sources of tryptophan, which serves as a basis for the creation of serotonin—one of the brain's primary mood-regulating neurotransmitters. Asparagus also boasts high levels of folate, a nutrient that may fight depression.

YOU'LL NEED

2 teaspoons extra-virgin olive oil

1 slice uncured turkey bacon, chopped

1 cup chopped asparagus

½ cup chopped zucchini

½ teaspoon minced garlic

¼ teaspoon crushed red pepper flakes

3 eggs, lightly beaten

Salt and black pepper, to taste

HOW TO MAKE IT

1. Heat the olive oil in a frying pan. Cook the bacon until crispy and remove from pan. Sauté the asparagus and the zucchini with the garlic and red pepper flakes until almost soft; set aside.

2. Add the eggs to pan and cook over medium-high heat, tilting the pan until egg sets. Add the bacon and zucchini/asparagus mixture to one-half of the omelet.

3. Fold the other half of the omelet over and transfer it to a plate. Add salt and pepper to taste.

KITCHEN SECRET: Use a spiralizer to turn zucchini into pasta, the perfect base for a fried egg.

Makes 1 serving
338 calories
27.8 g fat (5.5 g saturated)
374 mg sodium
8.8 g carbs
3.6 g fiber
4.6 g sugar
26.4 g protein

EAT CLEAN, EAT BEAN OMELET

Why shell out your hard-earned dollars for an overpriced gut bomb when you can make something better, healthier, and cheaper at home in ten minutes flat? This averages out to about $1.50 per serving.

YOU'LL NEED

One 14–16-ounce can black beans, drained

Juice of 1 lime

¼ teaspoon cumin

Hot sauce

Nonstick cooking spray, butter, or olive oil, for greasing the pan

8 eggs

Salt and black pepper to taste

½ cup feta cheese, plus more for serving

Bottled salsa

Sliced avocado (optional)

HOW TO MAKE IT

1. Pulse the black beans, lime juice, cumin, and a few shakes of hot sauce in the bowl of a food processor until it has the consistency of refried beans, adding a bit of water to help if necessary.

2. Coat a small nonstick pan with nonstick cooking spray and heat over medium heat. Crack 2 eggs into a bowl and beat with a bit of salt and pepper. Add the eggs to the pan, then use a spatula to stir and then lift the cooked egg on the bottom to allow the raw egg to slide under. When the eggs have all but set, spoon a quarter of the black bean mixture and 2 tablespoons of feta down the middle of the omelet. Use the spatula to fold over a third of the egg to cover the mixture in the center, then carefully slide the omelet onto a plate, using the spatula to flip it over at the last second to form one fully rolled omelet.

3. Repeat with the remaining ingredients to make four omelets. Garnish with salsa, avocado slices if you like, and a bit more crumbled feta.

Makes 4 servings.
Calculated without avocado
slices and salsa
517 calories
14.2 g fat (5.9 g saturated)
338 mg sodium
64.3 g carbs
15.1 g fiber
3.7 g sugar
35.2 g protein

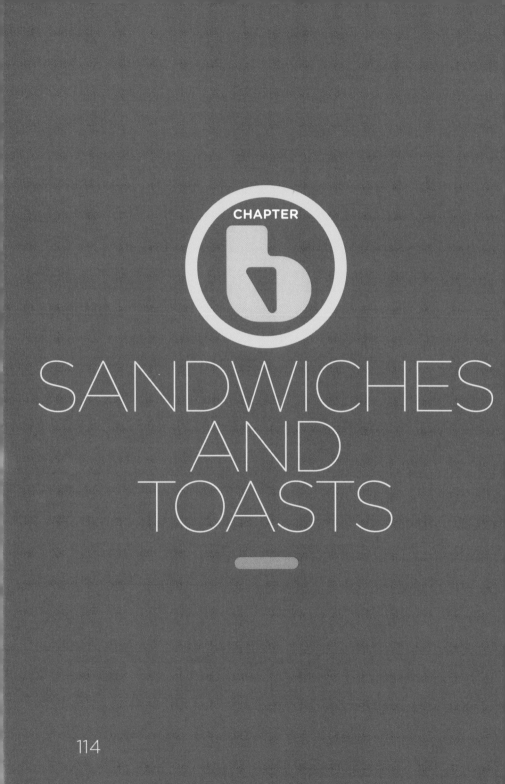

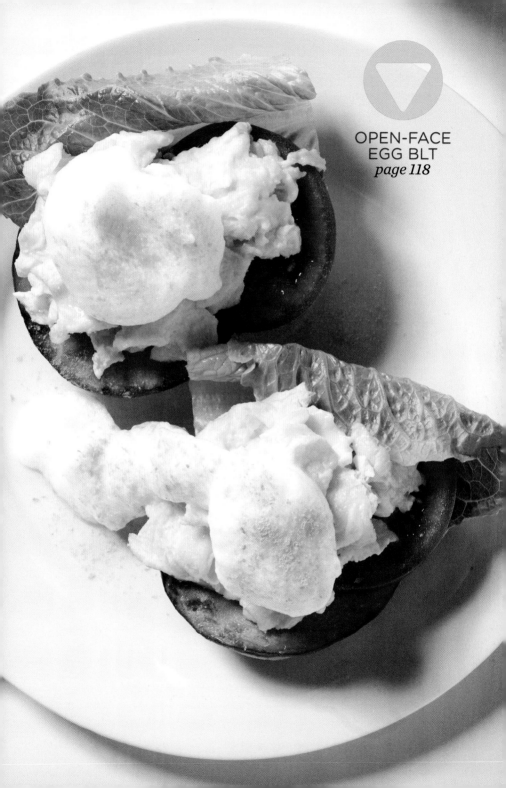

OPEN-FACE
EGG BLT
page 118

The more you think about the breakfast sandwich, the more glorious it becomes.

That soft, pillowy egg; that crispy, salty meat; that gooey, melty cheese; all perfectly nestled between the doughy goodness of toasted bread. It makes you believe all is right with the world. And yet, when you start to dissect what's actually in most breakfast sandwiches—creepy additives, a boatload of salt, and enough cholesterol to make an artery stiffen in fear—you start to wonder where the morning went all wrong.

A breakfast sandwich ought to be a no-brainer: Studies show that fueling up with a healthy combination of protein and whole grains can dull hunger and prevent weight gain. So the next time you get the urge to wrap your hands around a portable breakfast treat, stick with these delicious recipes, which include a selection of yummy toasts, too.

SMOKIN' SALMON SANDWICH

The New York classic—minus the bagel.

YOU'LL NEED

¼ cup **Tofutti cream cheese**

8 slices **gluten-free bread,** toasted

2 tablespoons **capers,** rinsed and chopped

½ **red onion,** thinly sliced

2 cups **mixed baby greens**

1 **large tomato,** sliced

Salt and black pepper, to taste

8 ounces **smoked salmon**

HOW TO MAKE IT

1. Spread 1 tablespoon of the cream cheese on each of four slices of toast. Top each with capers, onion, greens, and tomato. Salt and pepper the tomato—adding extra pepper. Finish by draping a few slices of smoked salmon over it.

Makes 4 sandwiches

315 calories
13.1 g fat (2.8 g saturated)
1,634 mg sodium
39.5 g carbs
5.7 g fiber
7.8 g sugar
14.3 g protein

OPEN-FACE EGG BLT

We've added eggs to this spin on the classic, for an extra 12 grams of protein.

YOU'LL NEED

1 teaspoon extra-virgin olive oil

1 gluten-free dinner roll, cut in half horizontally

2 slices uncured Canadian bacon

2 eggs, lightly beaten

Romaine lettuce

2 slices tomato

½ cup frothed aquafaba (see page 188)

½ teaspoon nutritional yeast

HOW TO MAKE IT

1. Heat the olive oil in the frying pan. Toast the roll with the cut sides down on the pan until golden while heating the Canadian bacon until lightly browned; set aside.

2. Scramble the eggs until desired doneness.

3. Divide evenly between each half roll and layer: Canadian bacon, lettuce, tomato, egg.

4. Top with aquafaba and sprinkle with nutritional yeast.

KITCHEN SECRET: This recipe also works with arugula, which goes great in an a.m. quinoa bowl too.

Makes 1 serving
Calculated without aquafaba
444 calories
25.6 g fat (4.7 g saturated)
709 mg sodium
32.8 g carbs
0.8 g fiber
1.5 g sugar
23.1 g protein

SRIRACHA EGG LETTUCE WRAP

Made from the paste of chili peppers, sriracha is literally the hottest condiment these days, in everything from potato chips and popcorn to jams and sauces. It's the perfect morning pick-me-up, especially since the capsaicin in the chili peppers has been proven to boost metabolism.

YOU'LL NEED

2 large lettuce leaves
(we used romaine, but iceberg may work better)

1 link chicken or turkey sausage
(we used organic sweet apple chicken sausage), heated and chopped

¼ **cup black beans**

¼ **cup chickpeas**

2 eggs, lightly beaten

¼ **cup tomatoes,** diced

Sriracha chili sauce
(we used about 2 teaspoons)

HOW TO MAKE IT

1. Place the lettuce leaves flat on a plate.

2. In a skillet over medium heat, brown the sausage.

3. Add the black beans and chickpeas, reduce the heat to low, and cook for 3 to 5 minutes; scoop even amounts onto the leaves.

4. Scramble the eggs to your liking and scoop even amounts over beans/sausage.

5. Top with tomatoes and sriracha.

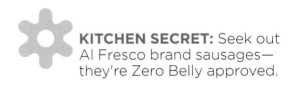

KITCHEN SECRET: Seek out Al Fresco brand sausages— they're Zero Belly approved.

Makes 1 serving
406 calories
10.6 g fat (13.1 g saturated)
696 mg sodium
50.5 g carbs
10.6 g fiber
3 g sugar
28.7 g protein

EGG SANDWICH
WITH PASTRAMI AND NOOCH

The combination of pastrami and Swiss has long been confined to the realm of the lunchtime deli counter, but we think it works beautifully with soft scrambled eggs—especially because pastrami trounces both sausage and bacon in the calorie department. Give it a try. Here, we swap the Swiss for nooch, a.k.a. nutritional yeast, for a dairy-free treat.

YOU'LL NEED

1½ teaspoons extra-virgin olive oil

4 ounces lean pastrami (or turkey pastrami), cut into strips

6 eggs

2 tablespoons almond milk

Salt and black pepper, to taste

2 tablespoons nutritional yeast

4 gluten-free English muffins, lightly toasted

HOW TO MAKE IT

1. Pour the olive oil in a large nonstick skillet over medium heat. Add the pastrami and sauté for 2 to 3 minutes. Reduce the heat to low. Combine the eggs with the milk and a few pinches of salt and pepper. Whisk lightly, then add to the pan. Use a wooden spoon to constantly stir the eggs, scraping from the bottom as they set, as they'll continue to cook once removed from the stovetop.

2. Spoon the nutritional yeast on each English muffin. Divide the scrambled eggs among the muffins, top with the muffin tops, and serve.

KITCHEN SECRET:
Pastrami has 6 grams of protein per slice, but it is salty. Enjoy responsibly.

Makes 4 servings
303 calories
12.2 g fat (3.8 g saturated)
743 mg sodium
28.6 g carbs
3.3 g fiber
3 g sugar
20.8 g protein

MASTER THE EGG

The Norma Desmond of breakfasts, the egg is the star and it deserves a bit of attention. If scrambling, use low heat and a constant stirring motion to create soft curds. If frying, cook the egg in extra-virgin olive oil over medium heat just until the white sets.

MAKE IT MOIST
Nobody wants a dry sandwich, and the same holds true in the morning hours. Salsa and hot sauce are the most obvious additions, but guacamole, pesto, and chimichurri all make incredible additions to the final package.

PACK ON THE PRODUCE
Most people think of breakfast sandwiches as meat-and-cheese affairs, but you should view them as the perfect opportunity to sneak some vegetation into your diet. Arugula adds a spicy kick, roasted bell peppers bring smoky sweetness, and avocado con-tributes fiber, healthy fat, and incredible richness to the table.

SUNNY-SIDE UP
AVOCADO
TOASTS
page 126

SUNNY-SIDE UP AVOCADO TOASTS

by Patricia Bannan, MS, RDN

Avocado toast is all the rage on Instagram and for good reason: No other fruit is credited with spot-reducing belly fat, warding off hunger, boosting nutrient absorption, lowering cholesterol, and fighting free radicals. They're best known for their high healthy fat content—9 percent!—and it's this richness of monounsaturated and oleic fatty acids that gives the amazing produce its viral-worthy status.

YOU'LL NEED

½ **large avocado,** mashed

2 large eggs

2 slices multigrain bread

¼ **teaspoon sea salt for sprinkling**

¼ **teaspoon red pepper flakes** (optional)

1 green onion, thinly sliced (optional)

1 radish, thinly sliced (optional)

HOW TO MAKE IT

1. In a small bowl, mash the avocado and set aside.

2. In a small skillet, fry each egg until your desired doneness. Meanwhile, toast the sliced bread. Add some mashed avocado to each toast, season with a pinch of sea salt and red pepper flakes, and top with a fried egg. If desired, garnish the toasts with a few sliced green onions, radishes, and another pinch of red pepper flakes. Serve right away.

Makes 2 servings
200 calories
11 g fat (2.5 g saturated)
418 mg sodium
4 g fiber
450 mg sodium
2.5 g sugar
10 g protein

Says Patricia: "It's super easy to make, tastes delicious, and is packed with protein and fiber to keep your hunger at bay until lunch—all for only 200 calories. You can season it as you like, adding red pepper flakes or even a splash of Sriracha sauce for a hot kick."

EGG & ONION RING ON AVOCADO TOAST

The rye and onion flavors evoke Zabar's, New York's classic Upper West Side gourmet grocery, known for its brunch staples.

YOU'LL NEED

1 slice gluten-free rye bread

¼ **cup avocado,** mashed

¼ **teaspoon garlic powder**

1 **teaspoon extra-virgin olive oil**

One ½-inch-thick slice from a 3-inch-diameter onion

1 **egg**

Pinch of crushed red pepper flakes

Salt and black pepper, to taste

HOW TO MAKE IT

1. Toast the rye bread.

2. Mix the avocado with garlic powder and spread on to toast.

3. Heat the oil in a small pan and add the onion slice; sauté 2 to 3 minutes on one side, then flip over.

4. Crack the egg into the center of the onion slice and cook for a few minutes until you see that the bottom of the egg is set.

5. Carefully flip over and cook the other side of the egg to your desired doneness.

6. Serve the egg ring on top of the avocado toast.

7. Sprinkle red pepper flakes, salt, and pepper to taste.

Makes 1 serving
253 calories
17.2 g fat (3.5 g saturated)
179 mg sodium
21.3 g carbs
5.2 g fiber
2.1 g sugar
7.5 g protein

COCONUT EGGS ON TOAST

by Stephanie Brookshier, RDN, ACSM-CPT

We're nuts for coconut oil, because it's a guaranteed metabolism booster. Studies show that the capric acid and other medium-chain triglycerides can increase 24-hour energy expenditure in humans by as much as 5 percent. That's an extra 100 to 120 calories per day!

YOU'LL NEED

3 large eggs

Dash of salt

Black pepper, to taste

2 teaspoons culinary coconut oil

½ avocado, sliced

2 slices gluten-free bread, toasted

Tomato (optional)

Chives (optional)

Parsley (optional)

Red pepper flakes (optional)

Cilantro (optional)

HOW TO MAKE IT

1. In a bowl, whisk together the eggs with the salt and pepper.

2. Heat a nonstick frying pan. Melt the coconut oil in the pan. Once the oil has melted and is clear, add the eggs.

3. Using a wooden spoon, stir gently, distributing all the runny parts of the egg so they scramble and cook evenly.

4. Use a fork to mash the avocado slices evenly onto the toast. Sprinkle with salt and pepper.

5. Top with the coconut-scrambled egg mixture.

6. Garnish with a tomato slice, chives, parsley, red pepper flakes, or cilantro if desired.

Makes 2 servings
329 calories
23.8 g fat (8.3 g saturated)
198 mg sodium
22.9 g carbs
8.4 g fiber
1.8 g sugar
13.4 g protein

Says Stephanie: "This quick dish has the right combination of protein, fat, and carbohydrates to keep you full until lunch and has fiber and prebiotics which are important for gut health. For a twist, switch up a slice of bread for a whole-wheat tortilla or two corn tortillas and add hot sauce."

TROPICAL TOAST & BERRIES

Ditch the sugary jam and top your toast with some fruit and dairy-free yogurt instead. This recipe takes just a few minutes to make yet still provides the nutrition you need to stay satisfied and full: complex carbs, fiber, and healthy fats.

YOU'LL NEED

2 slices of sprouted-grain bread

¼ cup plain dairy-free yogurt

1 teaspoon honey

½ cup fresh berries

1 teaspoon unsweetened coconut flakes

Cinnamon, to taste

HOW TO MAKE IT

1. Toast the bread. While the bread is toasting, mix together the yogurt and honey in a small bowl. After you've removed the bread from the toaster, spread the yogurt mixture on each slice of toast. Then top with the berries, coconut flakes, and cinnamon.

KITCHEN SECRET: Raspberries contain anthocyanins, a naturally occurring class of chemicals that increase insulin and lower blood sugar levels, warding off diabetes.

Makes 1 serving
191 calories
3 g fat (1.5 g saturated)
103 mg sodium
6.5 g fiber
13 g sugar
7 g protein

SHROOM FOR TWO BREAKFAST CUPS

Eggs served over toast—amazing. Eggs on mushroom caps? Even better. Swap in your favorite veggies to make these breakfast cups all your own. There's no end to limit the combinations you can create.

YOU'LL NEED

2 large portobello mushrooms, stems removed

3 teaspoons extra-virgin olive oil

¼ **large onion,** chopped

½ **bell pepper,** chopped

1 clove garlic, finely chopped

½ **cup spinach,** chopped

1 small turkey sausage, sliced

Salt and black pepper, to taste

2 eggs

2 small slices of avocado

HOW TO MAKE IT

1. Put the portobello caps on a rimmed baking sheet and drizzle with 1½ teaspoons of olive oil. Broil for about 12 minutes, or until tender. Meanwhile, heat the remaining 1½ teaspoons of olive oil in a skillet over medium heat. Add the onion, bell pepper, and garlic to the skillet and cook until fragrant. Then, add the spinach and turkey sausage. Season with salt and black pepper, reduce the heat to low, cover with a lid, and cook for 5 minutes more.

2. While the vegetables finish cooking, fry the eggs, sunny-side up, over medium heat. Top the cooked portobellos with the sautéed vegetables and avocado slices, then add the egg on top.

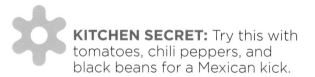

KITCHEN SECRET: Try this with tomatoes, chili peppers, and black beans for a Mexican kick.

Makes 2 servings
227 calories
16 g fat (3.5 g saturated)
266 mg sodium
2 g fiber
3 g sugar
11.5 g protein

THE BREAKFAST SANDWICH MATRIX

Start with an egg. Reams of research have shown that moderate consumption of eggs has no negative effect on cholesterol, and some argue they may boost good cholesterol.

Choose Your Style of Egg

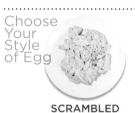

SCRAMBLED

Choose Your Protein

> Want perfect bacon every time? Bake in a 375°F oven for 15 minutes.

BACON   **HAM**   **TURKEY**

Choose Your Produce

> Fresh baby spinach and wilted spinach are both excellent with fried or scrambled eggs.

AVOCADO   **TOMATO**   **SPINACH**

Choose Your Add-ons

SALSA   **GUACAMOLE**   **SRIRACHA/HOT SAUCE**

Choose Your Vessel

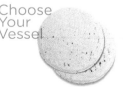

CORN TORTILLAS   **GLUTEN-FREE WRAP**   **GLUTEN-FREE ENGLISH MUFFIN**

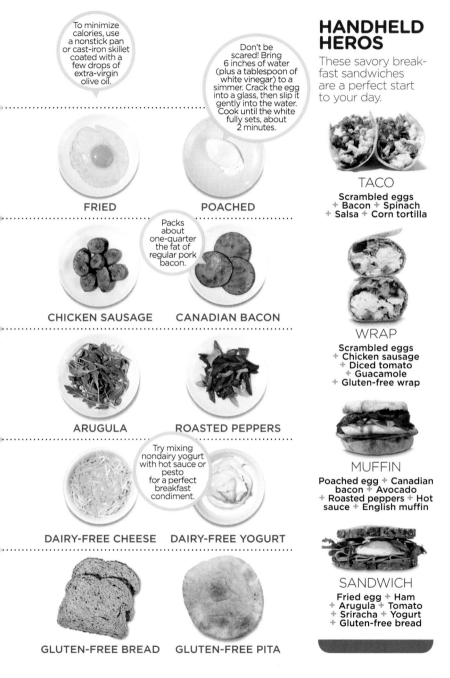

To minimize calories, use a nonstick pan or cast-iron skillet coated with a few drops of extra-virgin olive oil.

Don't be scared! Bring 6 inches of water (plus a tablespoon of white vinegar) to a simmer. Crack the egg into a glass, then slip it gently into the water. Cook until the white fully sets, about 2 minutes.

HANDHELD HEROS

These savory breakfast sandwiches are a perfect start to your day.

FRIED

POACHED

TACO
**Scrambled eggs
+ Bacon + Spinach
+ Salsa + Corn tortilla**

Packs about one-quarter the fat of regular pork bacon.

CHICKEN SAUSAGE

CANADIAN BACON

WRAP
**Scrambled eggs
+ Chicken sausage
+ Diced tomato
+ Guacamole
+ Gluten-free wrap**

ARUGULA

ROASTED PEPPERS

MUFFIN
**Poached egg + Canadian
bacon + Avocado
+ Roasted peppers + Hot
sauce + English muffin**

Try mixing nondairy yogurt with hot sauce or pesto for a perfect breakfast condiment.

DAIRY-FREE CHEESE

DAIRY-FREE YOGURT

SANDWICH
**Fried egg + Ham
+ Arugula + Tomato
+ Sriracha + Yogurt
+ Gluten-free bread**

GLUTEN-FREE BREAD

GLUTEN-FREE PITA

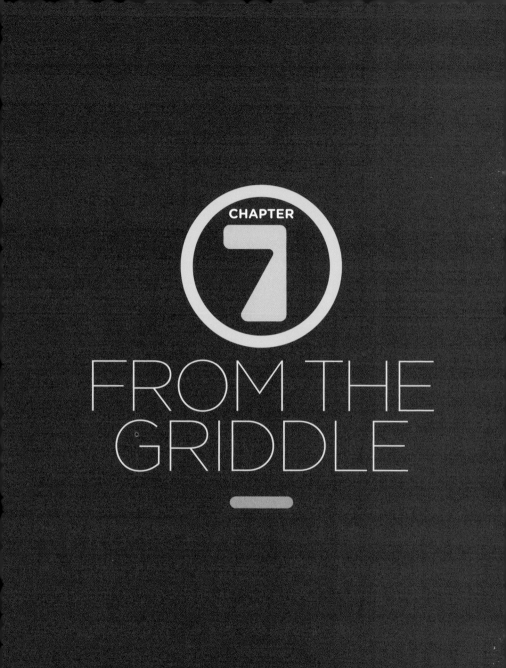

CHAPTER

7

FROM THE
GRIDDLE

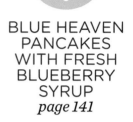

BLUE HEAVEN
PANCAKES
WITH FRESH
BLUEBERRY
SYRUP
page 141

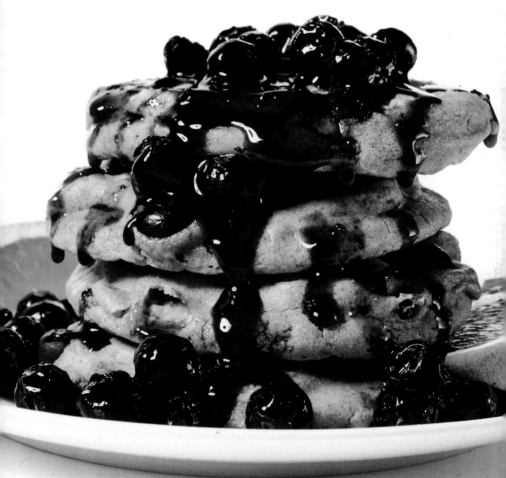

hen I set out to create Zero Belly Diet, I had two things in mind: 1) Making sure you'll lose weight safely, effortlessly, and quickly, armed with the latest science that targets your belly fat first and 2) pancakes. You gotta be allowed to eat pancakes.

This chapter is the culmination of all that hard work.

It wasn't easy. Zero Belly Diet is mainly gluten-free and dairy-free—and wheat and milk are two key ingredients in most griddle recipes. Not to mention, a tree-full of maple syrup isn't exactly allowed on any diet. (Most of the recipes in this book are free from added sugars.)

Despite these constraints, the master chefs in the Zero Belly test kitchen developed these mouthwatering recipes. And the result is a diet without the bait and switch.

That happens over and over with diet plans—they seem simple enough to follow at first, but then they start promising you that your waffle craving can be suppressed with a handful of veggies, or that drinking a glass of water will make you completely forget your craving for French toast. Instead of tricking and depriving yourself, why not swap some of the unhealthy ingredients for more protein, fiber, and flavor? On Zero Belly Diet, you can have your pancakes and eat them, too.

BLUE HEAVEN PANCAKES
WITH FRESH BLUEBERRY SYRUP

The breakfast staple—now guilt-free.

YOU'LL NEED

SYRUP

¼ cup fresh blueberries

2 tablespoons maple syrup

2 tablespoons water

PANCAKES

2 cups oat flour

1 tablespoon baking powder

¼ teaspoon kosher salt

1 cup unsweetened almond milk

1½ teaspoons extra-virgin olive oil

1 egg

½ teaspoon vanilla extract

Juice of ½ lemon

2 egg whites, whipped to soft peaks

Olive oil spray

½ cup fresh blueberries

BLUE HEAVEN PANCAKES WITH FRESH BLUEBERRY SYRUP
continuation

HOW TO MAKE IT

1. Prepare the syrup. Combine the blueberries, maple syrup, and water in a small saucepan and place it over medium heat. Bring to a low simmer and cook for 5 minutes, stirring occasionally. Set aside.

2. Heat a griddle or a large cast-iron pan over medium heat.

3. In a bowl, mix together the flour, baking powder, and salt.

4. In a separate bowl, whisk together the almond milk, olive oil, egg, vanilla, and lemon juice.

5. Combine the wet and dry ingredients and mix until just combined. Gently fold in the egg whites.

6. Lightly coat the griddle or cast-iron pan with olive oil spray and use a 2-ounce ladle or a ¼-cup measure to ladle the pancakes onto the pan.

7. Cook for about 2 minutes on the first side. Just before flipping, top with a few blueberries. Flip the pancake with a heatproof spatula and cook for 1 to 2 minutes more. Repeat with remaining batter, for about 12 pancakes total.

8. Divide the pancakes among four plates (three per plate) and top with a spoonful of the blueberry syrup.

Makes 4 servings
(12 pancakes)
261 calories
7 g fat
35 g carb
7 g fiber
11 g protein

10-MINUTE BREAKFAST

QUICKIE WAFFLES WITH HAM & EGG

YOU'LL NEED

Olive oil cooking spray
1 slice Canadian bacon
1 egg
1 Van's gluten-free waffle

Pepper, to taste
1 tablespoon nutritional yeast
Parsley (optional)

HOW TO MAKE IT

1. Heat a nonstick skillet or sauté pan over medium heat. Coat with a bit of olive oil cooking spray and cook the Canadian bacon for a few minutes on each side, until well browned. Remove. Coat the same pan with a bit more spray and cook the egg.

2. In the meantime, toast the waffle. Top it with a slice of meat and the warm egg. Season with pepper and nutritional yeast and sprinkle with parsley if using.

Makes 1 serving
270 calories
11 g fat (3.5 g saturated)
33 g carbs
9 g fiber
890 mg sodium
26 g protein

FLOURLESS BANANA PANCAKES

by Leah Kaufman, MS, RD, CDN, of Leah Kaufman Nutrition

Almond butter has more heart-healthy monounsaturated fatty acids than peanut butter, and it's just as convenient. It's amazing the way it holds these pancakes together.

YOU'LL NEED

1 banana

2 tablespoons almond butter

1 egg

Dash of cinnamon

Dash of nutmeg

Nonstick cooking spray

1 teaspoon maple syrup as desired

HOW TO MAKE IT

1. Mash the banana and almond butter together.

2. In a separate bowl, beat the egg. Combine the ingredients and add the cinnamon and nutmeg for flavor.

3. Spray the pan with nonstick cooking spray. Add half the mixture and cook over low heat until golden brown on bottom. Flip the pancake and cook until cooked through. Repeat with remaining mixture.

4. Add maple syrup as desired and enjoy!

Says Leah: "This recipe is great as it uses minimal ingredients, yet is a perfect combination of fruit, protein, and healthy fats. It is quick and easy to prepare before heading out the door."

*Makes 1 serving
(two pancakes)*
384 calories
22.9 g fat (3 g saturated)
65 mg sodium
38.6 g carbs
6.5 g fiber
20.2 g sugar
13.7 g protein

PUMPKIN-LATTE PANCAKES
WITH APPLE BUTTER

Because pumpkin spice lattes were made to be eaten.

YOU'LL NEED

2 cups gluten-free flour blend (we prefer Pillsbury)

6 tablespoons brown sugar

2 teaspoons baking powder

2 teaspoons pumpkin pie spice

½ teaspoon sea salt

¾ cup canned pumpkin puree

4 large eggs

½ cup unsweetened applesauce

⅔ cup unsweetened almond milk

1 tablespoon canola or vegetable oil, plus more as needed

Apple butter (no high-fructose corn syrup) **or pure maple syrup**

HOW TO MAKE IT

1. Preheat the oven to 350°F.

2. In a large bowl, whisk together the flour, brown sugar, baking powder, pumpkin pie spice, and salt.

3. In a medium bowl, whisk together the pumpkin puree, eggs, applesauce, and almond milk.

4. Gently stir the wet ingredients into the dry ingredients just until combined. The batter will be thick.

5. Heat the vegetable oil in a large nonstick skillet over medium heat. Using ⅓ cup of batter for each pancake, cook until the edges firm up and the bottom is golden brown, about 1½ minutes. Flip and cook until the other side is golden brown, about 1½ minutes. Place on a large rimmed baking sheet. Cook the remaining batter, transferring the pancakes in a single layer to the baking sheet when done, adding more oil to the pan as needed.

6. Bake the pancakes for an additional 5 minutes to finish cooking. Serve with apple butter or maple syrup.

Makes 4 servings
Calculated without apple
butter or maple syrup
421 calories
9.8 g fat (2.5 g saturated)
345 mg sodium
70.6 g carbs
3.8 g fiber
18.3 g sugar
13.5 g protein

CRISPY VEGGIE PANCAKES
WITH BASIL-CURRY MAYO

A savory breakfast pancake? Sweet!

YOU'LL NEED

1 medium zucchini, shredded

1½ pounds russet potatoes, peeled and shredded

1 large carrot, peeled and shredded

¼ cup gluten-free flour blend (we prefer Pillsbury)

1 large egg, beaten

**2 teaspoons snipped fresh thyme,
 or ½ teaspoon dried thyme**

½ teaspoon salt, plus more for seasoning

¼ teaspoon freshly ground black pepper,
 plus more for seasoning

2 tablespoons canola or vegetable oil

½ cup gluten-free mayonnaise

2 tablespoons finely snipped fresh basil

1½ teaspoons curry powder

½ teaspoon smoked paprika

Thinly sliced green onions

HOW TO MAKE IT

1. Preheat the oven to 200°F.

2. Place the zucchini in a colander. Press firmly to squeeze out as much excess liquid as possible. In a large bowl, combine the zucchini, potatoes, carrot, flour, egg, thyme, salt, and pepper.

3. Heat 1 tablespoon of the canola oil in an extra-large nonstick skillet over medium heat. For each pancake, spoon about ½ cup of the potato mixture into the skillet. Evenly press and round the edges with the back of a spatula to form pancakes. Cook for 4 to 5 minutes on each side, until golden brown and crisp. Transfer the pancakes to a large rimmed baking sheet and keep warm while cooking the remaining pancakes in the remaining oil.

4. In a small bowl, stir together the mayonnaise, basil, curry powder, and paprika. Season to taste with salt and pepper.

5. Top the pancakes with a dollop of curry mayonnaise and green onions.

Makes 4 servings
257 calories
9.7 g fat (2 g saturated)
348 mg sodium
37.6 g carbs
6 g fiber
4 g sugar
6.3 g protein

BUCKWHEAT PANCAKES WITH CHERRY COMPOTE

Every ½-cup serving of buckwheat packs 3 grams of protein, 2 grams of belly-flattening fiber, and half the day's magnesium. Now in pancake form.

YOU'LL NEED

One 14-ounce can red tart cherries in water, drained

1 tablespoon sugar

2 tablespoons water

1 teaspoon lemon zest

1 small cinnamon stick

½ cup gluten-free flour blend (we prefer Pillsbury)

⅓ cup buckwheat flour

¾ teaspoon baking soda

¼ teaspoon salt

1 tablespoon brown sugar

1¼ cups plain unsweetened almond milk

4 tablespoons canola or vegetable oil

1 large egg

HOW TO MAKE IT

1. Preheat oven to 200°F.

2. For the compote, combine the cherries, sugar, water, lemon zest, and cinnamon stick in a medium saucepan. Bring to a low boil over medium heat. Reduce the heat to a simmer. Cover and cook for about 8 minutes, until slightly thickened.

3. Meanwhile, in a medium bowl, whisk together the gluten-free flour, buckwheat flour, baking soda, salt, and brown sugar.

4. In another medium bowl, whisk together the almond milk, 3 tablespoons of the canola oil, and the egg until well blended.

5. Gently stir the wet ingredients into the dry ingredients just until blended.

6. Heat the remaining tablespoon of oil in a large nonstick skillet over medium-high heat. For each pancake, spoon a scant ¼ cup of batter into the skillet, spreading the batter lightly with the back of a spoon. Cook until bubbles form on the surface of the pancakes, about 2 minutes. Flip and cook 1 to 2 minutes more. Transfer to a rimmed baking sheet and keep warm in the oven while cooking the remaining pancakes.

7. Serve the pancakes topped with compote.

Makes 2 servings
(a serving is 1 pancake)
375 calories
16.5 g fat (3.3 g saturated)
476 mg sodium
52.3 g fiber
2.4 g fiber
5.6 g sugar
5.1 protein

CHOCOLATE-BANANA WAFFLES

Yes: Chocolate. Banana. Waffles.

YOU'LL NEED

2 cups gluten-free flour blend (we prefer Pillsbury)

½ cup unsweetened cocoa

¼ cup sugar

½ teaspoon salt

1 tablespoon baking powder

½ teaspoon cinnamon

2 eggs

One 14-ounce can full-fat coconut milk

1 ripe banana, thoroughly mashed

1 teaspoon vanilla extract

1 teaspoon dairy-free chocolate-hazelnut butter (we prefer Justin's)

1 banana, sliced

1 ounce chopped toasted hazelnuts

CHOCOLATE-
BANANA WAFFLES

CHOCOLATE-BANANA WAFFLES
continuation

HOW TO MAKE IT

1. In a large bowl, whisk together the flour, cocoa, sugar, salt, baking powder, and cinnamon.

2. In a medium bowl, whisk the eggs, coconut milk, banana, and vanilla.

3. Gently stir the wet ingredients into the dry ingredients just until combined.

4. Cook in a waffle iron according to the manufacturer's instructions.

5. Top with chocolate-hazelnut butter, banana slices, and hazelnuts.

Makes 4 servings
476 calories
12.2 g fat (4.2 g saturated)
330 mg sodium
84.5 g carbs
8.3 g fiber
22.1 g sugar
13.3 g protein

KITCHEN SECRET

SPECIAL SAUCE

While we've managed to take most of the sting out of the French toast, it's still by definition a carb-heavy breakfast. But by increasing your fiber intake, you can blunt the impact on your blood sugar levels. Try replacing the syrup with any of the following:

- Sliced bananas, either raw or caramelized in a pan over medium heat for a few minutes

- Blueberries cooked for 15 minutes with a spoonful of water

- Raw strawberries with powdered sugar

SAVORY FRENCH TOAST

Recent studies have shown that garlic supports blood sugar metabolism and helps control lipid (fat) levels in the blood. Bonus: Adding garlic to foods that are rich in fats and carbohydrates may keep those substances from doing the damage they're known to do.

YOU'LL NEED

2 large eggs

⅓ cup plus 2 tablespoons plain unsweetened almond milk

2 cloves garlic, minced

Pinch crushed red pepper flakes

2 tablespoons minced fresh parsley, plus additional for garnish

Salt and black pepper, to taste

2 tablespoons extra-virgin olive oil

4 slices gluten-free bread

½ cup sugar-free marinara sauce, warmed

2 tablespoons green onions, finely sliced

HOW TO MAKE IT

1. Preheat the oven to 200°F.

2. In a large bowl, whisk together the eggs, almond milk, garlic, red pepper flakes, parsley, and salt and black pepper to taste.

3. Heat 1 tablespoon of olive oil in a large skillet over medium heat. Swirl to coat. Dip one slice of bread in the egg mixture. Lay in the skillet. Repeat with another piece of bread. Cook, swirling the pan occasionally, for about 8 minutes total, until deep golden brown on both sides. Transfer to a plate and keep warm in the oven while cooking the remaining bread in the remaining olive oil.

4. Serve topped with warm marinara and sprinkled with green onions and additional parsley.

Makes 2 servings
Calculated with ½ cup
marinara sauce
311 calories
22.1 g fat (4.2 g saturated)
494 mg sodium
20.3 g carbs
2.7 g fiber
6.9 g sugar
9.4 g protein

APRICOT-JACKPOT FRENCH TOAST

Besides flushing out extra water weight, potassium—found in apricots—also keeps your metabolism running high and is crucial for the digestion of carbs and fat.

YOU'LL NEED

¾ cup all-fruit apricot preserves (no sugar or high-fructose corn syrup)

¼ cup snipped dried apricots

¼ cup chopped walnuts

Two 4-ounce loaves gluten-free French-style baguettes (we prefer Udi's)

2 large eggs

½ cup plain unsweetened almond milk

¼ teaspoon ground nutmeg

¼ teaspoon vanilla extract

1 tablespoon canola or vegetable oil

2 tablespoons orange juice

Fresh raspberries

HOW TO MAKE IT

1. Preheat the oven to 300°F.

2. For the filling, in a small bowl, combine ¼ cup of the preserves, dried apricots, and walnuts; set aside.

3. Cut the bread into 1½-inch-thick slices. Cut a pocket in the top of each bread slice, being careful not to cut all the way to the sides. Divide the filling evenly among the bread slices.

4. In a medium bowl, whisk the eggs, almond milk, nutmeg, and vanilla. Heat the canola oil in large non-stick skillet over medium heat. Using tongs, quickly dip the filled bread slices in the egg mixture, allowing any excess mixture to drip off (take care not to squeeze out the filling). Cook for about 4 minutes, until golden brown, turning once. Transfer to a rimmed baking sheet and keep warm in the oven while cooking the remaining slices.

5. Meanwhile, in a small saucepan, combine the remaining ½ cup of apricot preserves and the orange juice; heat and stir until the mixture is melted.

6. To serve, drizzle the hot French toast with the preserves. Top with raspberries.

Makes 4 servings

414 calories
13.7 g fat (1.8 g saturated)
403 mg sodium
67.3 g carbs
3.9 g fiber
29.6 g sugar
10.7 g protein

VANILLA-BOURBON FRENCH TOAST

The French call this *pain perdu,* "lost bread," a nod to the fact that it works best with stale bread. The French also serve *pain perdu* as a dessert, a reminder that this dish is traditionally soaked in sugar and cream! This version forgoes cream for milk, and a deluge of sugar for vanilla and a slug of bourbon. Good morning indeed.

YOU'LL NEED

4 eggs

1½ cups almond milk

¼ cup bourbon

1 teaspoon vanilla extract

1 tablespoon sugar

¼ teaspoon ground nutmeg

1 loaf day-old country bread, preferably whole-wheat, cut into 8 slices

Extra-virgin olive oil, for the pan

Maple or agave syrup, for serving

Powdered sugar, for dusting (optional)

HOW TO MAKE IT

1. Preheat the oven to 225°F.

2. Combine the eggs, almond milk, bourbon, vanilla, sugar, and nutmeg in a shallow baking dish and whisk to combine. Soak each slice of bread for 30 seconds, turning once, before cooking.

3. Heat a large cast-iron skillet or nonstick pan over medium heat. Pour olive oil in the pan. Add 2 to 4 slices of the soaked bread and cook for about 3 minutes, until a deep brown crust forms. Flip the bread and continue cooking for 2 to 3 minutes more, until golden brown and firm to the touch. Keep the cooked French toast in the oven while you work through the rest of the batch.

4. Serve with warm syrup and a dusting of powdered sugar, if you like.

Makes 4 servings

340 calories
10.5 g fat (3.8 g saturated)
416 mg sodium
40.6 g carbs
4.2 g fiber
18.4 g sugar
13.2 g protein

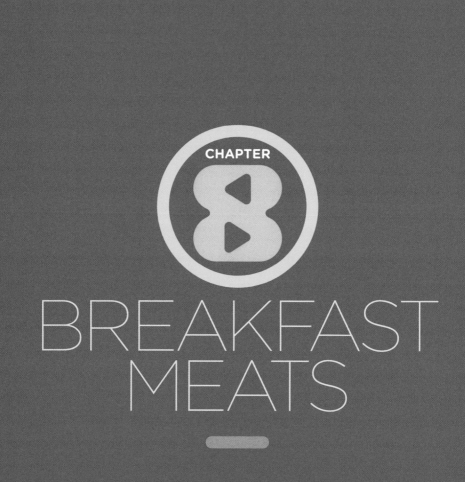

CHAPTER

8

BREAKFAST
MEATS

STEAK &
EGGS WITH
CHIMICHURRI
page 165

Not too many people know this, but the B in Zero Belly stands for "bacon."

Okay, that's not actually true—it stands for beans and healthy fibers. But it's no secret that bacon makes everything better. The recipes in this chapter include pork of all varieties, as well as chicken and turkey, each high in fiber, healthy fats, and protein. That last point's key.

Among nutrients, protein has the best publicist in the world—news about its importance in your diet is everywhere. But unlike other faddish foods—dietary Kardashians, if you will—it deserves all the hype. Protein is essential not just for bulking your biceps but for revving your metabolism, boosting your brainpower, trimming your middle, and generally realizing your flat-belly goals. You should make it a goal for protein to play a starring role in each meal. But you don't have to scarf protein shakes or chase chickens like Wile E. Coyote to get enough. On Zero Belly Diet, you'll find diverse, surprising options to enjoy at any time of day, from breakfast to snack time to before bed. After all, bacon makes everything better—especially diets.

THE HANGOVER CURE

STEAK & EGGS
WITH CHIMICHURRI

There's nothing subtle about the commingling of seared steak and egg yolk in the morning. You know you're in for something serious even before it hits the table. Amazingly enough, though, this is a near-perfect nutritional start to your day, loaded with protein, healthy fat, and even a bit of fiber. This meal works as well at 11:30 a.m., as a cure for a hangover or post-workout hunger pangs, as it does at 8 p.m., as a remedy for a long day at work.

KITCHEN SECRET: Grass-fed beef is naturally leaner and has fewer calories than conventional meat, and some cuts have more omega-3s than salmon.

STEAK & EGGS WITH CHIMICHURRI
continuation

YOU'LL NEED

FOR THE CHIMICHURRI

1 cup coarsely chopped parsley (about half a bunch)

1 clove garlic

½ teaspoon salt

2 tablespoons water

1½ tablespoon red wine vinegar

¼ cup extra-virgin olive oil

½ teaspoon sugar

1 tablespoon minced jalapeño

FOR THE STEAK AND EGGS

1 tablespoon olive oil

1 pound flank or skirt steak

Salt and black pepper, to taste

4 Roma tomatoes, halved lengthwise

4 eggs

HOW TO MAKE IT

1. CHIMICHURRI: Combine all of the ingredients in the bowl of a food processor and pulse until fully blended. Makes about 1 cup; keeps in the refrigerator for up to 1 week.

2. STEAK & EGGS: Heat 1½ teaspoons of the olive oil in a grill pan or cast-iron skillet over high heat. Season the steak all over with salt and pepper. Cook, turning the steak every minute or so, for 7 to 8 minutes total, until fully browned on the outside and firm but fully yielding to the touch. Remove to a cutting board and rest for 5 minutes before slicing.

3. While the steak rests, place the tomatoes cut-side down in the same pan and cook for about 2 minutes, until the bottoms are lightly blackened.

4. Heat the remaining 1½ teaspoons of the olive oil in a large nonstick pan. Working in batches, crack the eggs into the pan and fry until sunny-side up, the whites just set and the yolks still loose. Season with salt and pepper.

5. Slice the steak against the natural grain of the meat. Divide the eggs and tomatoes among four warm plates. Spoon the chimichurri liberally over the steak and eggs.

Makes 4 servings
382 calories
26.6 g fat (6.4 g saturated)
363 mg sodium
5.6 g carbs
1.6 g fiber
3.4 g sugar
29.9 g protein

CHIMICHURRI

This bright green garlic and parsley sauce is Argentina's most ubiquitous condiment for a reason: It has that unique power to make almost everything taste better. Grilled steak and chimi is the classic combo, but it makes even more sense when you add eggs to the picture. Beyond beef, try chimichurri as a sandwich spread, as a topping for roast chicken or grilled fish, or as a dipping sauce for grilled asparagus or crispy roasted potatoes. It keeps for a week in the fridge and gets better with time, so make up a big batch and go to town.

BACON & EGG NESTS

Bacon's great, just don't pig out.

YOU'LL NEED

8 slices Canadian bacon, chopped

4 green onions, sliced

One 10.7-ounce package sweet potato "noodles"

½ teaspoon kosher salt

1 teaspoon black pepper

2 tablespoons extra-virgin olive oil

4 eggs

HOW TO MAKE IT

1. Preheat the oven to 425°F. In a large skillet, cook the bacon over medium heat until crisp. Remove from the skillet and drain on paper towels.

2. Place the green onions, vegetable noodles, salt, and pepper on a rimmed baking sheet. Drizzle with olive oil; toss gently to combine. Roast for 30 to 35 minutes or until noodles are tender, gently stirring once or twice.

3. Make four nests or indentations in the noodles, about 2 inches apart. Carefully crack one egg into each nest. Roast for 8 to 10 minutes more, or to desired doneness. Sprinkle with bacon.

Makes 4 servings
463 calories
16.7 g fat
(4.1 g saturated)
648 mg sodium
66.4 g carbs
6.5 g fiber
0.7 g sugar
10.6 protein

OVEN-ROASTED TURKEY SAUSAGE
WITH GARLIC-TURMERIC SWEET POTATOES

by Jim White, RDN, of Jim White Fitness and Nutrition Studios

Creating your own patties, rather than buying store brands, cuts the sodium in half.

YOU'LL NEED

16 ounces ground turkey sausage

2 sweet potatoes

2 cloves garlic, minced

SEASONING FOR POTATOES

1 tablespoon black pepper

½ tablespoon garlic powder

1 tablespoon lemon juice

1 tablespoon turmeric

HOW TO MAKE IT

1. Preheat the oven to 425°F.

2. Make the turkey sausage into 4 equal-size patties.

3. Peel the sweet potatoes and cut them into 2-inch cubes. Place the potatoes in a deep bowl. Add the pepper, garlic powder, lemon juice, and turmeric. After each potato piece is covered in seasoning mix, put them in an 8 x 9-inch pan with edges.

4. Take the patties out of the refrigerator and place them next to the sweet potatoes. Top with minced garlic. Place in the oven for 45 minutes (be sure the potatoes are soft and the patties are cooked thoroughly).

Makes 4 servings
468 calories
32.5 g fat (10.4 g saturated)
856 mg sodium
19.6 g carbs
3.3 g fiber
0.7 g sugar
23.5 g protein

Says Jim: "Turkey sausages are a great swap for pork sausages. It is much lower in calories and fat, while still providing you with 23 grams of protein per 4-ounce patty. The turmeric in the potato seasoning blend offers a powerful natural anti-inflammatory and antioxidant, and sweet potatoes are packed with vitamins and minerals, which is great to start your day with."

SMOKED SALMON, AVOCADO, & ARUGULA BREAKFAST SALAD

Yes, you read that right—this is a salad for breakfast. This special type of salad has all the traditional makings of a healthy bowl of greens but infuses it with traditional morning staples like smoked salmon and eggs. Give it a try; we know you'll love it!

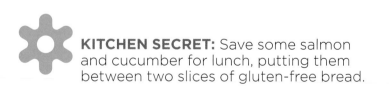

KITCHEN SECRET: Save some salmon and cucumber for lunch, putting them between two slices of gluten-free bread.

YOU'LL NEED

1½ **cups arugula,** washed and dried

¼ **avocado,** sliced

¼ **cucumber,** sliced

2 ounces smoked salmon, sliced

1 egg, hard-boiled, sliced in half

1½ **teaspoons sesame seeds**

Juice from ¼ **lime**

1½ **teaspoons extra-virgin olive oil**

Salt, to taste

HOW TO MAKE IT

1. In a salad bowl, combine the arugula, avocado, cucumber, salmon, and egg.

2. Top with sesame seeds, lime juice, olive oil, and salt to taste, and toss well to combine the flavors.

Makes 1 serving
341 calories
26 g fat (5.3 g saturated)
1,000 mg sodium
5.5 g fiber
3 g sugar
19 g protein

SAUSAGE, EGG, & AVOCADO BREAKFAST BOWL

Think of this as a breakfast burrito bowl. By combining all of the delicious things you'd find inside a hearty morning wrap— but ditching the doughy carb blanket— you get a tasty meal that's low-cal and hits all of the nutritional marks.

YOU'LL NEED

2 large turkey sausage links, sliced

4 eggs, hard-boiled, peeled, and cut into fourths

1½ cups cherry tomatoes, halved

2 tablespoons red onion, chopped

½ avocado, diced

¼ cup fresh cilantro, chopped

Salt and black pepper, to taste

Juice of 1 lemon

HOW TO MAKE IT

1. Start by cooking the sausage according to the package instructions. After they've cooked through, set them aside on a paper towel.

2. In a large bowl, combine the sausage, eggs, tomatoes, onion, avocado, cilantro, salt, pepper, and lemon juice. Stir with a large spoon until the egg yolks and avocado start to create a creamy texture.

KITCHEN SECRET: Hold the Pepto-Bismol and garnish your meals with cilantro. Research shows the herb's unique blend of oils works like over-the-counter meds to relax digestive muscles.

Makes 2 servings
310 calories
22 g fat (6 g saturated)
379 mg sodium
14 g carbs
6 g fiber
6 g sugar
16 g protein

SAUTÉED CINNAMON- SAGE APPLES
WITH COTTAGE BACON

Cottage bacon is made from the pork shoulder, not the belly, and, as a result, it's leaner but no less crispy.

YOU'LL NEED

3 teaspoons canola or vegetable oil

4 ounces cottage bacon or Canadian bacon, chopped

2 large Granny Smith apples, peeled, cored, and sliced

¼ teaspoon apple pie spice or cinnamon

½ to 1 teaspoon snipped fresh sage

Pure maple syrup

HOW TO MAKE IT

1. Heat 1 teaspoon canola oil in a large skillet over medium heat. Cook the bacon, stirring, for 3 to 5 minutes, until lightly browned. Remove the bacon from skillet with a slotted spoon; set aside.

2. Heat the remaining 2 teaspoons of oil in the skillet over medium-high heat. Add the apples to the skillet. Sprinkle with the apple pie spice and sage. Cook for 4 to 5 minutes, until apples are golden brown.

3. Stir in the bacon and warm through. Serve with maple syrup.

KITCHEN SECRET: A series of studies printed in the *American Journal of Clinical Nutrition* found that adding a heaping teaspoon of cinnamon to a starchy meal may help stabilize blood sugar and ward off insulin spikes, keeping you away from the snack drawer hours longer.

Makes 2 servings
319 calories
11.2 g fat (2.6 g saturated)
803 mg sodium
45.4 g carbs
5.5 g fiber
35.1 sugar
12.3 g protein

CHORIZO & POTATO HASH
WITH EGGS

The pork sausage turns chicken in this healthier, gluten-free twist.

YOU'LL NEED

2 large russet potatoes, peeled and cut into ½-inch dice

1 tablespoon distilled white vinegar

1 tablespoon kosher salt

2 tablespoons extra-virgin olive oil

1 medium sweet onion, chopped

2 cloves garlic, minced

3 links fully cooked gluten-free chicken chorizo (we prefer Aidell's), cut into ¼-inch-thick slices

4 large eggs

Salt and black pepper, to taste

Snipped fresh cilantro or parsley

Salsa verde (optional)

HOW TO MAKE IT

1. Preheat the oven to 375°F.

2. Place the potatoes in a medium saucepan and cover with cold water. Add the vinegar and salt. Bring to a boil; reduce the heat to a simmer and cook for 5 minutes, or until the potatoes are barely tender. Drain the potatoes in a colander for at least 5 minutes. (This step can be done ahead; the potatoes can be stored in a sealed container in the refrigerator for up to 3 days.)

3. Meanwhile, in a large oven-proof skillet, heat 1 table-spoon olive oil over medium heat. Add the onion and garlic and cook for 3 to 4 minutes, until beginning to soften. Add the chorizo slices and cook for 3 to 4 minutes, until browned and crisp.

4. Remove the sausage and onion mixture from the skillet with a slotted spoon; set aside. Heat the re-maining tablespoon of olive oil in the skillet over medium-high heat. Cook the potatoes for 3 to 5 minutes, until lightly browned and crisp, stirring occa-sionally. Add the sausage and onion mixture back to the skillet. Stir to combine.

5. Make four shallow wells in the potato mixture. Crack an egg into each well. Bake for 8 to 10 minutes, or until the whites are set but the yolks are still runny. Season with salt and pepper to taste. Sprinkle with cilantro or parsley. Serve with salsa, if desired.

Makes 4 servings
318 calories
14.7 g fat (3.4 g saturated)
270 mg sodium
32.5 g carbs
5 g fiber
3.7 g sugar
14.8 g protein

CRISPY CAJUN CHICKEN TENDERS
WITH GREEN ONION GRITS

Go to bed in your house. Wake up to a N'awlins Mardi Gras in your mouth.

YOU'LL NEED

Olive oil spray, if using

¾ cup gluten-free flour blend
(we prefer Pillsbury)

2 teaspoons Cajun seasoning blend

¾ teaspoon salt

Black pepper

1 large egg

1 pound chicken tenders

⅓ cup yellow cornmeal

1 cup quick-cooking grits

¼ cup sliced green onions

Hot sauce

Makes 4 servings
387 calories
10.6 g fat (2.8 g saturated)
670 mg sodium
32.1 g carbs
2.6 g fiber
1.1 g sugar
38.4 g protein

HOW TO MAKE IT

1. Preheat the oven to 425°F. Line a rimmed baking sheet with parchment paper (or spray with olive oil spray).

2. Place 3 medium bowls in a row. In bowl #1, combine ½ cup gluten-free flour blend, 1 teaspoon Cajun seasoning, ¼ teaspoon of the salt, and pepper to taste. Whisk to combine.

3. Beat the egg in bowl #2.

4. In bowl #3, combine the remaining ¼ cup of gluten-free flour blend, the cornmeal, the remaining 1 teaspoon of Cajun seasoning, ¼ teaspoon of the salt, and pepper to taste. Whisk to combine.

5. Dredge each chicken tender in the mixture in bowl #1, coating completely and shaking off any excess. Dip in beaten egg, then dip in the cornmeal mixture in bowl #3, pressing to coat completely. Place on the prepared baking sheet. Repeat with remaining chicken tenders.

6. Bake in the oven for 12 to 14 minutes, turning once, until cooked through and golden brown.

7. Meanwhile, heat 4 cups water to boiling in a large saucepan. Gradually whisk the grits and the remaining ¼ teaspoon of salt into the water. Reduce the heat to medium-low; cover. Cook for 5 to 7 minutes or until thick, stirring occasionally. Remove from the heat. Stir in the onions and pepper to taste, and serve the tenders with grits and hot sauce.

CHICKEN SAUSAGE
WITH POLENTA, ZUCCHINI, & PEPPERS

Polenta, a resistant starch, takes a while to digest, keeping you fuller, longer.

YOU'LL NEED

¼ **cup sun-dried tomatoes,** snipped

1 cup plain unsweetened almond milk

1 cup gluten-free, reduced-sodium chicken broth

½ **cup yellow cornmeal** (polenta)

Salt and black pepper

1 tablespoon extra-virgin olive oil

2 fully cooked gluten- and dairy-free Italian-style chicken-turkey sausages (we prefer Applegate) or chicken-apple sausage links, cut into ¼-inch-thick slices

½ **small onion,** thinly sliced

1 small zucchini or yellow summer squash, thinly sliced

½ **small red or yellow bell pepper,** cut into strips

Snipped fresh parsley

HOW TO MAKE IT

1. In a small bowl, cover the sun-dried tomatoes with boiling water; set aside. In a medium saucepan, combine almond milk and chicken broth. Bring just to boiling over high heat. Gradually whisk in the cornmeal. Reduce the heat to medium-low. Cook, stirring frequently, for 12 to 15 minutes, until thick and creamy. Season to taste with salt and black pepper. Reduce the heat to low; cover and keep warm.

2. Meanwhile, drain the tomatoes. In a large skillet, heat the olive oil. Brown the sausage slices in the hot oil for 2 to 3 minutes. Add the tomatoes, onion, zucchini, and bell pepper to the pan. Cook, stirring occasionally, for 3 to 5 minutes or until tender. Season to taste with salt and black pepper.

3. To serve, ladle the polenta into two shallow bowls. Top with the sausage-zucchini mixture. Sprinkle with parsley.

Makes 2 servings
298 calories
22 g fat (5.2 g saturated)
1,073 mg sodium
11.2 g carbs
2.2 g fiber
6.4 g sugar
17.4 g protein

CHICKEN-FRIED STEAK & GRAVY
WITH FRIZZLED EGGS

The Wiener Schnitzel of the South is a bit high in calories—but protein, too.

YOU'LL NEED

1 8-ounce rib-eye steak, cut about ½ inch thick

Salt and black pepper

½ cup gluten-free flour blend (we prefer Pillsbury)

¼ cup plain unsweetened almond milk

2 teaspoons hot pepper sauce

3 tablespoons canola or vegetable oil

1 clove garlic, minced

1 cup gluten-free beef broth

2 teaspoons cornstarch

1 teaspoon snipped fresh thyme,
   or ¼ teaspoon dried thyme

2 large eggs

Snipped fresh thyme
   (optional)

Makes 2 servings
585 calories
39.6 g fat (12.4 g saturated)
434 mg sodium
25.8 g carbs
1.2 g fiber
1 g sugar
32.1 g protein

HOW TO MAKE IT

1. Trim the fat from the steak. Cut in half crosswise to make two portions. Place each portion on a piece of plastic wrap. Using the tenderizing side of a meat mallet, pound each steak lightly until about ¼ inch thick. Season with salt and pepper to taste.

2. Place the flour in a shallow dish. In another shallow dish, combine the almond milk and hot pepper sauce. Dip the steaks in the flour, turning to coat and shaking off any excess. Dip into the almond milk mixture, then in the flour again, turning to coat.

3. In a medium skillet, heat 2 tablespoons canola oil over medium-high heat. Add the steaks; cook for 5 to 6 minutes or until golden, turning once. Transfer the steaks to a serving platter, reserving the drippings from the skillet. Cover the steaks and keep warm.

4. For the gravy, add the garlic to the pan and briefly cook for 1 minute. Add the broth to the pan, scraping up the browned bits. Bring to a simmer. In small bowl or cup, combine the cornstarch with 1 tablespoon cold water. Slowly pour the mixture into the hot broth, whisking constantly. Simmer, whisking occasionally, for 2 to 3 minutes, until thickened. Whisk in the thyme. Cover and keep warm.

5. For the frizzled eggs, in a medium skillet, heat the remaining tablespoon of oil over medium-high heat. When the oil is hot, crack the eggs into the skillet. Cook until the edges of the eggs are browned and crisp and the yolks are the desired doneness.

6. Top the steaks with the gravy and serve with the eggs. Sprinkle with fresh thyme, if desired.

BREAKFAST CHOPS
WITH SWEET POTATO HASH BROWNS

Save this one for a big Sunday brunch.
Served best when eaten with a lumberjack.

YOU'LL NEED

½ **pound sweet potato**
(about half of a large sweet potato),
peeled and grated

2 teaspoons snipped fresh chives

Salt and black pepper

3 tablespoons canola or vegetable oil,
plus additional if needed

2 pork breakfast chops*

¼ **teaspoon dried thyme**

⅛ **teaspoon garlic powder**

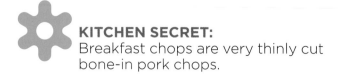

KITCHEN SECRET:
Breakfast chops are very thinly cut
bone-in pork chops.

HOW TO MAKE IT

1. Preheat the oven to 200°F. Line a rimmed baking sheet with paper towels.

2. Place the grated potatoes in a clean kitchen towel or three layers of 100% cotton cheesecloth. Twist the cloth to squeeze out as much moisture as possible. In a medium bowl, combine potatoes and chives. Season to taste with salt and pepper. Toss to combine.

3. In a large skillet, heat 2 tablespoons of the canola oil over medium heat. When the oil is hot, scoop large spoonfuls of sweet potatoes into the pan, forming small mounds. Use a spatula to gently press and spread the mounds slightly. Cook for about 4 to 5 minutes, until nicely browned on one side. Carefully flip over with a metal spatula and cook on the other side for 4 to 5 minutes. Place on a rimmed baking sheet and keep warm in the oven.

4. Season the chops with thyme, garlic powder, salt, and pepper. In the same skillet, heat the remaining tablespoon of oil over medium-high heat. Cook the chops for 2 to 3 minutes, until browned. Flip and cook 1 to 2 minutes more, until cooked through.

5. Serve the chops with the hash browns.

Makes 2 servings
480 calories
33.7 g fat (10.1 g saturated)
97 mg sodium
23.7 g carbs
3.9 g fiber
7.4 g sugar
20.3 g protein

SIDES AND SAUCES

① ROASTED GARLIC

When roasted until sweet and nutty, garlic has more in common with butter than it does with the raw, pungent stuff we're all used to. Use a few cloves to spike mayonnaise or to enhance a salad dressing.

YOU'LL NEED

1 head garlic   **1½ teaspoons extra-virgin olive oil**

HOW TO MAKE IT

1. Preheat the oven to 400°F.

2. Use a knife to cut off the top ¼ inch of the garlic head, barely exposing the top part of the individual cloves. Place the garlic in the center of a piece of aluminum foil and drizzle the olive oil on top. Cover the garlic with the foil and fold the ends to create a sealed packet, then place in the oven and roast for 35 to 40 minutes, until very soft. Keeps in the fridge for up to a week.

Makes 1 head

② AQUAFABA

This vegan meringue was an Internet sensation—its very name was crowdsourced, combining the Latin for water and the Latin for bean, and reversing it. Use it instead of mayo for any recipe.

YOU'LL NEED

One 15-ounce can chickpeas

HOW TO MAKE IT

1. Using the liquid from one can of chickpeas—just use the liquid, set the beans aside or store for another use—mix with an electric mixer for about 10 minutes, or until frothy.

Makes about 1 cup

3 PICKLED JALAPEÑOS

Don't limit these chilies to dinner; try them on breakfast sandwiches and omelets—or anything that would benefit from a sharp, spicy-sweet kick.

YOU'LL NEED

8 to 10 jalapeños
1 cup rice wine or cider vinegar
1 cup water

1 tablespoon salt
1 tablespoon sugar

HOW TO MAKE IT

1. Cut the jalapeños into thin slices. If you like your peppers hot, cut all the way up to the stem; for a milder batch, stop ½ inch before.

2. Combine the vinegar, water, salt, and sugar in a saucepan and heat just enough so that the salt and sugar dissolve. Allow the liquid to cool briefly.

3. Place the jalapeños in a sterilized jar or small mixing bowl. Pour the liquid over them, then cover, letting them soak for at least 10 minutes before using. Will keep for 1 week covered in the refrigerator.

Makes about 2 cups

4 PICO DE GALLO

The most versatile of all salsas, this chunky mix is delicious.

YOU'LL NEED

4 Roma tomatoes, chopped
1 small red onion, diced
1 jalapeño, minced

1 handful cilantro, chopped
Juice of 1 lime
Salt and black pepper, to taste

HOW TO MAKE IT

1. Combine the tomatoes, onion, jalapeño, cilantro, and lime juice in a mixing bowl. Season with salt and pepper and mix to thoroughly combine. Keeps covered in the refrigerator for up to 1 week.

Makes about 3 cups

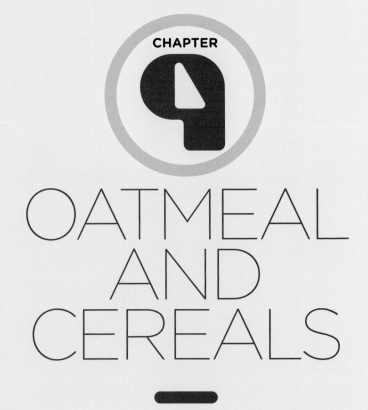

CHAPTER

9

OATMEAL AND CEREALS

—

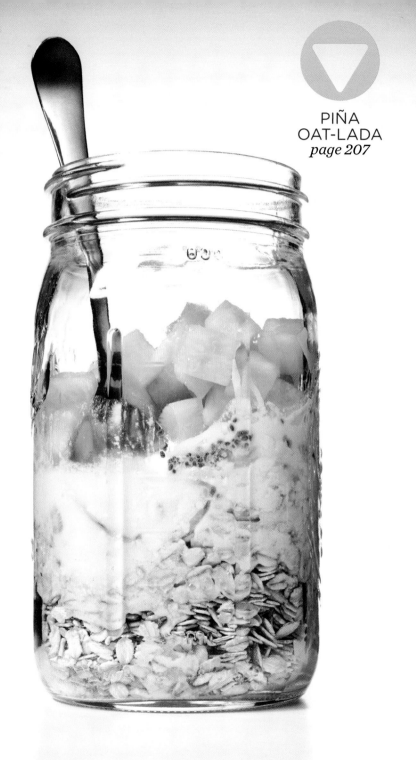

PIÑA
OAT-LADA
page 207

We've discovered a magical food that helps you lose weight, lower your cholesterol, and reduce your risk of type 2 diabetes for as little as 13 cents per day. And you've probably got a tub of it in your kitchen right now.

There are some big reasons why little old oatmeal is such a power player: Not only is it packed with fiber, a nutrient that accelerates weight loss, it's also one of the very best sources of resistant starch. That's the kind that digests slowly and triggers the release of digestive acids that suppress appetite and accelerate calorie burn. In fact, one study found that swapping just 5 percent of daily carbohydrates for resistant starch could boost your metabolism by a whopping 23 percent!

Here, we've mixed it with the best Zero Belly fruits and mix-ins, threw in some fun cereals, too, and added a special section on Overnight Oats. Because what's better than a meal for 13 cents a day? A meal you don't have to cook.

BLACKBERRY PIE

With 7.6 grams of fiber per cup, blackberries are one of the best high-fiber foods.

YOU'LL NEED

½ **cup unsweetened almond milk**

½ **cup water**

½ **cup rolled oats**

½ **cup blackberries**

1 tablespoon raw flaked almonds

1 teaspoon chia seeds

Dash of cinnamon

HOW TO MAKE IT

1. Bring the almond milk and water to a boil in a saucepan. Stir in the oats and cook for about 3 minutes, until soft.

2. Just before the oats are finished, remove from the heat and stir in the blackberries. Top with the almonds, chia seeds, and cinnamon.

Makes 1 serving

239 calories
7.6 g fat (0.8 g saturated)
93 mg sodium
37.5 g carbs
9.7 g fiber
4.1 g sugar
8.2 g protein

BUCKWHEAT
WITH PEA PROTEIN

Like quinoa, buckwheat is gluten-free and a complete source of protein, meaning it supplies all nine essential muscle-building amino acids the body cannot produce on its own.

YOU'LL NEED

¼ **cup dry cream of buckwheat**

1 cup almond milk, vanilla unsweetened

1 scoop plain pea protein

1 tablespoon agave syrup

1 teaspoon cinnamon

½ **banana,** mashed

1 tablespoon dairy-free dark chocolate chips

Berries (optional)

HOW TO MAKE IT

1. Prepare buckwheat: Mix the buckwheat with ¾ cup almond milk and heat in the microwave for about 3 minutes.

2. Mix the pea protein into the remaining ¼ cup of almond milk and mix into the hot cream of buckwheat.

3. Stir in the agave, cinnamon, and banana.

4. Top with chocolate chips. Add the berries for extra nutrition, if using.

KITCHEN SECRET: Blend the pea protein into the almond milk and then cook your oats for even more protein.

Makes 1 serving
Calculated without berries
407 calories
5.7 g fat (1.3 g saturated)
375 mg sodium
74.6 g carbs
4.7 g fiber
11.3 g sugar
20.2 g protein

COCONUT BERRY BLAST OATMEAL

by Jim White, RDN, of Jim White Fitness and Nutrition Studios

Berries are a staple of Zero Belly Diet. Here, you get three kinds—and coconut!

YOU'LL NEED

2 cups unsweetened coconut milk

1 cup old-fashioned oatmeal

2 teaspoons raw honey

1 cup blended blueberries, strawberries, and raspberries

1 teaspoon flaxseeds

1 teaspoon chia seeds

1 tablespoon shredded coconut

HOW TO MAKE IT

1. Mix together the coconut milk, oatmeal, and honey in a saucepan and bring to a boil, then reduce the heat and simmer for about 10 minutes until fully cooked.

2. In the bowl of a blender, blend together the fruit, flaxseeds, and chia seeds until smooth.

3. Stir the berry blend into the oatmeal mixture.

4. Serve hot (leftovers can be refrigerated and warmed up or eaten cold). Top with coconut.

Makes 1 serving
141 calories
4.3 g fat (2.6 g saturated)
2 mg sodium
23.6 g carbs
3.9 g fiber
6.8 g sugar
3.3 g protein

Says Jim: "This oatmeal is a great way to jump-start your day. The berry blend has a high content of antioxidant to protect the body from free radicals harmful to our body. The chia and flaxseeds contain omega-3 fatty acids, which are a good fat our body needs. The raw honey is great for a natural sweetener."

BERRY GOOD QUINOA
BREAKFAST SALAD

BERRY GOOD QUINOA BREAKFAST SALAD

Though quinoa isn't traditionally thought of as a breakfast carb, we think it ought to be. In this recipe it plays a starring role, along with fruit and nuts, to create a dish that's as colorful as a bowl of Lucky Charms—but free of the eerie chemicals. Another win: The primary components of this recipe are all filled with antioxidants that kill off health-harming free radicals.

Makes 3 servings
354 calories
11.7 g fat (1 g saturated)
6 mg sodium
52.7 g carbs
8.7 g fiber
9.6 g sugar
12.2 g protein

BERRY GOOD QUINOA BREAKFAST SALAD
continuation

YOU'LL NEED

FOR THE SALAD

1 cup quinoa, cooked and cooled

¾ **cup strawberries,** sliced in half

½ **cup raspberries**

½ **cup blueberries**

½ **cup raw almonds,** finely chopped

1½ **teaspoons mint,** finely chopped

1½ **teaspoons basil,** finely chopped

FOR THE DRESSING

½ **teaspoon orange zest**

2 tablespoons fresh orange juice

1 tablespoon fresh lemon juice

½ **tablespoon fresh lime juice**

1½ **teaspoons honey**

½ **teaspoon mint,** finely chopped

½ **teaspoon basil,** finely chopped

HOW TO MAKE IT

1. In a large bowl, combine all of the salad ingredients.

2. Then, in a separate bowl or jar, whisk together all of the dressing ingredients. Drizzle the desired amount over the salad mixture.

CHOCO-OATS

With a touch of chocolate, and tangy red berries, this is dessert for breakfast.

YOU'LL NEED

½ **cup rolled oats**

¾ **cup unsweetened coconut milk**

1 sliced banana

1½ **tablespoons unsweetened cocoa powder**

¼ **teaspoon coconut oil**

Colorful red berries as desired

HOW TO MAKE IT

1. Mix the oats, coconut milk, banana, cocoa powder, and coconut oil together in a saucepan and cook over medium to high heat for 6 minutes. Top with the berries.

Makes 1 serving
Calculated without berries
322 calories
8.3 g fat (5.2 g saturated)
5 mg sodium
60.5 g carbs
10.6 g fiber
15 g sugar
8.3 g protein

HOMEMADE COOKIE CRISP

I've been eating healthy for two decades, but whenever I see a commercial for Cookie Crisp, I can't help but howl like that cartoon dog. This version is for cheat days only.

YOU'LL NEED

FOR THE "COOKIE CRISP"

1 cup gluten-free flour

1 cup rolled oats

¾ teaspoon baking powder

½ teaspoon baking soda

½ teaspoon salt

⅓ cup coconut oil

1 extra-large egg

1 teaspoon vanilla extract

½ cup sugar

½ cup unsweetened dark chocolate chips

Nonstick spray

FOR SERVING THE CEREAL

1 cup almond milk

½ cup vanilla plant-based protein powder

HOW TO MAKE IT

1. Preheat the oven to 375°F.

2. Combine the flour, oats, baking powder, baking soda, and salt in a large mixing bowl. In a separate mixing bowl, beat the coconut oil, egg, vanilla, and sugar until you have a uniform consistency. Add the flour mixture to the bowl, mixing gently to combine. Mix in the chocolate chips.

3. Cover a cookie sheet with nonstick spray. Drop the dough on the sheet in small teaspoons. Bake for 7 minutes, just until the edges of the cookies begin to brown. Cool for a few minutes.

4. When cool, place a few small cookies in a bowl, add the milk, and stir in the protein powder.

KITCHEN SECRET: Easily the worst way to start your day, Honey Smacks is 60 percent flat-out sugar.

Makes about 42 Cookie Crisp-size cookies
Per bowl: 399 calories
21 g fat (15 g saturated)
645 mg sodium
14 g carbs
3.1 g fiber
15 g sugar
16.3 g protein

BANANA BREAD CHIA PUDDING

by Willow Jarosh & Stephanie Clarke, C&J Nutrition

Say Willow and Stephanie: "Craving banana bread? Put the baking dishes away and opt for this nutritious way to get your fix. Chia seeds are hydrophilic, meaning they can absorb much more liquid than their tiny size might indicate. That means that they keep you hydrated for a while after eating them and they also keep you feeling full and satisfied for longer. And because it's prepped ahead of time, it means we can be well fueled on super busy mornings."

YOU'LL NEED

3½ cups unsweetened dairy alternative milk (soy, almond, cashew, hemp, etc.)

3 very ripe bananas, mashed

½ cup chia seeds

2 teaspoons vanilla extract

1 teaspoon ground cinnamon

4 tablespoons chopped walnuts

HOW TO MAKE IT

1. Whisk the milk, bananas, chia seeds, vanilla, and cinnamon together. Cover with plastic wrap and refrigerate overnight.

2. Stir the pudding, divide it among 4 bowls, and top each serving with 1 tablespoon walnuts.

Makes 4 servings
Calculated with unsweetened
almond milk
222 calories
12.5 g fat (1 g saturated)
136 mg sodium
29.2 g carbs
8.9 g fiber
11.2 g sugar
6.6 g protein

OVERNIGHT OATS!

No time? No problem. Fill a Mason jar or Tupperware container with oats, toppings, add-ins, and a liquid such as milk or water. Then throw it in the refrigerator overnight. While you're sleeping, the flavors fuse together so all you have to do is scarf it down the next morning—no stovetop required!

YOU'LL NEED

1 cup oatmeal

1 cup plant-based milk of your choice

1 teaspoon chia seeds

1 Mason jar

½ scoop plant-based protein (optional)

HOW TO MAKE IT

Combine all of the ingredients in a Mason jar. Close the jar. Refrigerate overnight or for at least 5 hours. It keeps for 4 days max.

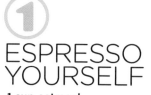

ESPRESSO YOURSELF

1 cup oatmeal
½ cup unsweetened coconut milk
½ cup of your favorite coffee
1 teaspoon chia seeds
1 teaspoon cocoa powder

Per bowl:
347 calories
8.4 g fat (3.1 g saturated)
8 mg sodium
58.4 g carbs
10.1 g fiber
0.8 g sugar
11.7 g protein

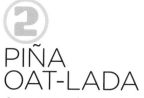

PIÑA OAT-LADA

1 cup oatmeal
1 cup unsweetened coconut milk
1 teaspoon chia seeds
⅓ cup shredded coconut
⅓ cup diced pineapple

Per bowl:
243 calories
9.6 g fat (6.4 g saturated)
5 mg sodium
34.8 g carbs
6.6 g fiber
4 g sugar
6.2 g protein

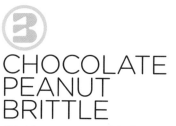

CHOCOLATE PEANUT BRITTLE

2 tablespoon peanut butter
   (without sugar)
1 cup oatmeal
1 cup unsweetened almond milk
1 teaspoon chia seeds
½ teaspoon vanilla extract
½ cup grated almonds
1 teaspoon unsweetened cocoa
   powder

Per bowl:
242 calories
12.2 g fat (1.6 g saturated)
104 mg sodium
27.3 g carbs
6.1 g fiber
1.4 g sugar
8.8 g protein

MATCHA MADE IN HEAVEN

1 cup oatmeal
1 cup unsweetened almond milk
1 teaspoon chia seeds
½ smashed banana
1 teaspoon matcha powder
Berries of your choice
   (for topping when serving)

Per bowl:
Calculated without berries
395 calories
9.8 g fat (1.4 g saturated)
186 mg sodium
71.9 g carbs
12.6 g fiber
8 g sugar
13.9 g protein

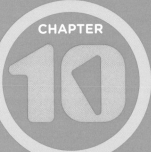

CHAPTER 10

ZERO BELLY SMOOTHIES

ALL SMOOTHIE RECIPES SERVE ONE.

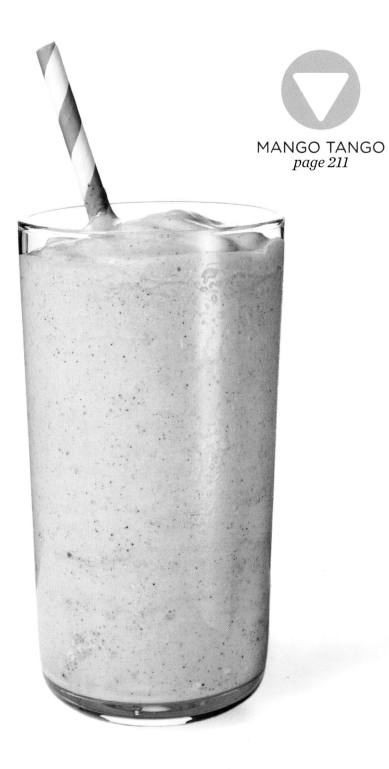

MANGO TANGO
page 211

A re you ready to lose weight with the press of a button? That's all it takes to blend up a Zero Belly Smoothie. I call it 60-second nutrition.

In every glass, you are getting a unique blend of supernutrients that help flatten your belly, boost your metabolism, and heal your digestive system. And the proof is in the results. I have seen test panelists lose up to 16 pounds in just 14 days with the Zero Belly Diet and the power of these smoothies—and they never felt hungry again.

How do they work? It's all about that base. Believe it or not, 65 percent of Americans are lactose intolerant, leading to bloat and poor digestion. Zero Belly Smoothies are made with nondairy milks such as unsweetened almond, cashew, or coconut milks, or green tea, which has zero calories!

And unlike most whey shakes, they're made with plant-based protein powder. Just last year, a major study from Harvard found that getting the majority of your protein from plant sources led to a lower risk of death compared to animal proteins.

Whip one up—and don't miss *Zero Belly Smoothies* for 100+ more recipes.

MANGO TANGO

The classic Indian Lassi gets a morning makeover, with 75 percent less sugar than the original—and all of the creamy, decadent flavor.

YOU'LL NEED

½ **cup mango**

1 frozen banana

1 cup unsweetened coconut milk

1 tablespoon cardamom

1 scoop vanilla plant-based protein powder

Water to blend (necessary)

HOW TO MAKE IT

1. Place all of the ingredients in the bowl of a blender and blend until smooth.

379 calories
6.9 g fat (4.8 g saturated)
464 mg sodium
66.9 g carbs
9.2 g fiber
44.4 g sugar
19.3 g protein

STRAWBERRY PISTACHIO CREAM

This one's a Test Panel Favorite from *Zero Belly Smoothies*. The Hulk-colored nuts have special fat-burning powers.

YOU'LL NEED

½ **cup frozen strawberries**

¼ **cup pistachios**

½ **avocado,** peeled, pitted, and quartered

3 ice cubes

1 teaspoon vanilla extract

1 scoop vanilla plant-based protein powder

Water to blend (necessary)

HOW TO MAKE IT

1. Place all of the ingredients in the bowl of a blender and blend until smooth.

266 calories
9 g fat (3 g saturated)
4 mg sodium
5 g fiber
8 g sugar
30 g protein

THE GREEN LIGHT

It may be green and leafy, but spinach is no nutritional wallflower. The muscle builder is a rich source of plant-based omega-3s and folate, which help reduce the risk of heart disease. All systems go.

YOU'LL NEED

1 frozen banana

1 handful of spinach

¼ cup pumpkin seeds

1 cup unsweetened almond milk

½ scoop vanilla plant-based protein powder

Water to blend (optional)

HOW TO MAKE IT

1. Place all of the ingredients in the bowl of a blender and blend until smooth.

388 calories
20.5 g fat (3.7 g saturated)
423 mg sodium
39.9 g carbs
6.1 g fiber
18.3 g sugar
19 g protein

SACHA FIERCE

Sacha inchi, a highly digestible superseed harvested from the Amazon, contains more omega-3s than any other seed on the planet, with 350 percent of the daily value. And now companies like Imlak'esh Organics (who provided this recipe) are bringing them mainstream.

YOU'LL NEED

1.5 ounces (or 2½ tablespoons) Imlak'esh Organics Sacha Inchi Protein Powder

¾ frozen banana

½ cup unsweetened cashew milk

½ cup sliced strawberries

1 tablespoon coconut blossom nectar (can substitute with honey)

½ to 1 cup of water

HOW TO MAKE IT

1. Place all of the ingredients in the bowl of a blender and blend until smooth.

345 calories
2.25 g fat (1 g saturated)
300 mg sodium
8.5 g fiber
12 g sugar
27 g protein

THE BRAIN BOOSTER!

CAFE OLÉ!

The secret ingredient here is magical: beans. Black beans are full of anthocyanins, anti-oxidant compounds that have been shown to improve brain function. You won't even taste them. And coffee, beyond boosting alertness for 90 minutes, is the #1 source of antioxidants in the American diet and can decrease your risk of Alzheimer's by as much as 60 percent.

YOU'LL NEED

1 cup frozen blueberries

¼ cup black beans

1 cup coffee

½ cup chocolate plant-based protein powder

2 ice cubes

HOW TO MAKE IT

1. Place all of the ingredients in the bowl of a blender and blend until smooth.

200 calories
9 g fat (3 g saturated)
300 mg sodium
3 g fiber
15 g sugar
22 g protein

ANTI-INFLAMMATORY TURMERIC PINEAPPLE SMOOTHIE

by Jennifer Cassetta, MS, CN, clinical nutritionist

Drink this if you have joint pain or arthritis, or if you are an athlete, to recover from a long day of hitting it hard.

YOU'LL NEED

½ cup coconut light milk

1 tablespoon coconut oil

½ cup frozen pineapple

½ banana

1 teaspoon turmeric

1 tablespoon hemp seeds

Handful of ice

½ cup water

HOW TO MAKE IT

1. Place all of the ingredients in the bowl of a blender and blend until smooth.

Says Jennifer: "This smoothie is chock-full of inflammation-fighting ingredients. Turmeric is a medicinal root that contains curcumin, which reduces inflammation naturally. Pineapple contains bromelain, also an anti-inflammatory agent. Hemp seeds contain omega-3 fatty acids that also reduce inflammation in the body."

234 calories
12 g fat (2 g saturated)
233 mg sodium
12 g fiber
7 g sugar
22 g protein

RED-LETTER DAY

Add four or five cubes, and you've got yourself an Italian cherry ice—in a glass.

YOU'LL NEED

½ **cup frozen strawberries**

½ **cup frozen cherries**

1 cup unsweetened coconut milk

½ **cup vanilla plant-based protein powder**

Ice cubes, to taste

HOW TO MAKE IT

1. Place all of the ingredients in the bowl of a blender and blend until smooth.

KITCHEN SECRET: Researchers have noted that cherry consumption has a profound ability to alter the expression of fat genes.

200 calories
9 g fat (3 g saturated)
300 mg sodium
3 g fiber
15 g sugar
22 g protein

THE SKIN SAVER!

ORANGE BLOSSOM

This one's made of carrots, oranges, turmeric, and sweet potatoes, giving it an orange glow. It's almost . . . presidential.

YOU'LL NEED

1 carrot

½ orange

½ tablespoon turmeric

1 cup unsweetened almond milk

½ cup plain plant-based protein powder

½ cup cooked sweet potato

2 ice cubes

HOW TO MAKE IT

1. Place all of the ingredients in the bowl of a blender and blend until smooth.

251 calories
6 g fat (2 g saturated)
295 mg sodium
3 g fiber
11 g sugar
22 g protein

THE ZERO BELLY SMOOTHIE MATRIX

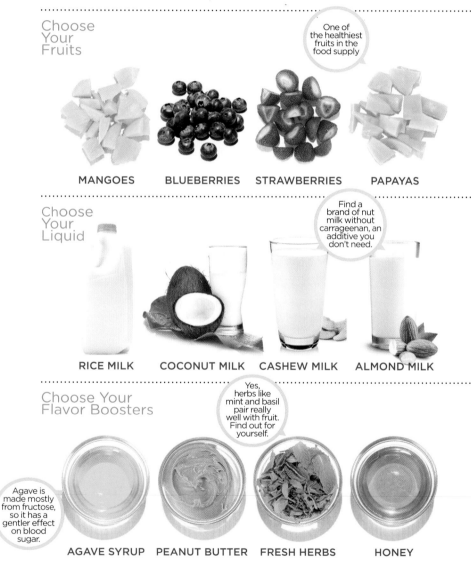

Choose Your Fruits

One of the healthiest fruits in the food supply

MANGOES   BLUEBERRIES   STRAWBERRIES   PAPAYAS

Choose Your Liquid

Find a brand of nut milk without carrageenan, an additive you don't need.

RICE MILK   COCONUT MILK   CASHEW MILK   ALMOND MILK

Choose Your Flavor Boosters

Yes, herbs like mint and basil pair really well with fruit. Find out for yourself.

Agave is made mostly from fructose, so it has a gentler effect on blood sugar.

AGAVE SYRUP   PEANUT BUTTER   FRESH HERBS   HONEY

Our recipes were developed by a team of dieticians, but you don't need a degree to create a healthy smoothie.

FANTASTIC FOUR

To the left are all the ingredients you need to custom blend your smoothies to ensure optimum performance.

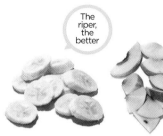

The riper, the better

BANANAS   PEACHES

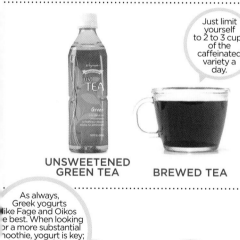

Just limit yourself to 2 to 3 cups of the caffeinated variety a day.

UNSWEETENED GREEN TEA   BREWED TEA

As always, Greek yogurts like Fage and Oikos are best. When looking for a more substantial smoothie, yogurt is key; just a cup of this stuff packs more than 15 grams of protein.

ALMOND YOGURT   VEGGIE PROTEIN

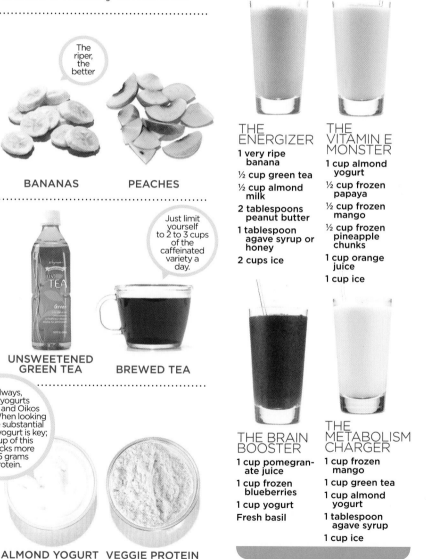

THE ENERGIZER

1 very ripe banana
½ cup green tea
½ cup almond milk
2 tablespoons peanut butter
1 tablespoon agave syrup or honey
2 cups ice

THE VITAMIN E MONSTER

1 cup almond yogurt
½ cup frozen papaya
½ cup frozen mango
½ cup frozen pineapple chunks
1 cup orange juice
1 cup ice

THE BRAIN BOOSTER

1 cup pomegranate juice
1 cup frozen blueberries
1 cup yogurt
Fresh basil

THE METABOLISM CHARGER

1 cup frozen mango
1 cup green tea
1 cup almond yogurt
1 tablespoon agave syrup
1 cup ice

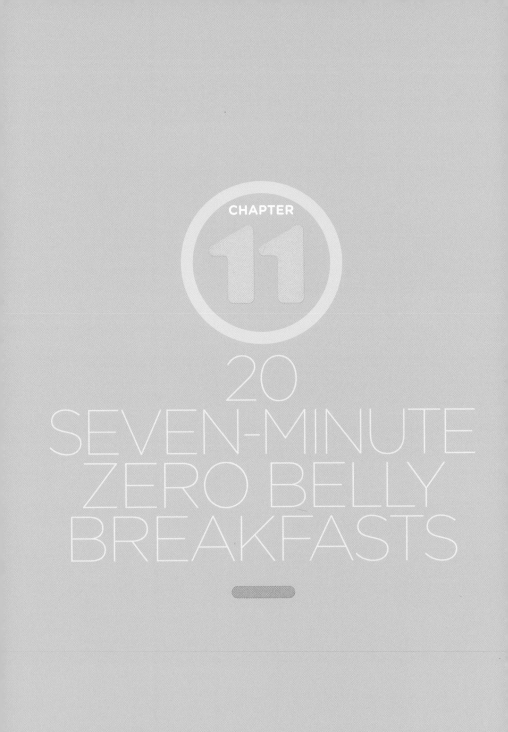

CHAPTER

11

20
SEVEN-MINUTE
ZERO BELLY
BREAKFASTS

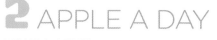

EGGS AND OMELETS

1 THE SEVEN-MINUTE OMELET

YOU'LL NEED

2 eggs
Handful of spinach

1 ounce smoked salmon
Spoonful of water

HOW TO MAKE IT

1. Heat a nonstick frying pan over medium-high heat. In a bowl, mix the eggs with a fork for 1 minute, adding the spinach and salmon as you mix. Pour the mixture into the frying pan. Let sit until the sides appear cooked and flaky. Pour the water into the pan and cover the pan with a lid. Let sit for 3 minutes, or until mixture looks cooked through. Remove from the heat, fold, and serve.

2 APPLE A DAY

YOU'LL NEED

2 eggs
1 teaspoon extra-virgin olive oil

½ apple
1 tablespoon almond butter

HOW TO MAKE IT

1. Heat a nonstick frying pan over medium-high heat. Add the olive oil. Crack the eggs into the pan and let cook until the egg whites are a bit firm, and then scramble with a fork in the pan. Cook until desired consistency is reached. Remove from the heat.

2. While the eggs cool, slice the apple and top with the almond butter. Serve with the eggs.

3 EGG AND SAUSAGE CUP

YOU'LL NEED

1 teaspoon olive oil
(for stovetop version)
2 eggs

½ Al Fresco–brand sausage, sliced
1 slice gluten-free bread

HOW TO MAKE IT

1. Microwave instructions: Whip the eggs for 1 minute and then pour them into a cup. Add the sausage. Cook on high for 40 seconds, and then remove and blend with a fork. Cook on high for another minute and serve.

2. Stovetop instructions: Heat a nonstick frying pan over medium-high heat. Add the olive oil. Crack the eggs into the pan and let cook until the egg whites are a bit firm, and then scramble them with a fork in the pan and add the sausage. Cook until desired consistency is reached. Remove from the heat.

3. Serve with toasted bread.

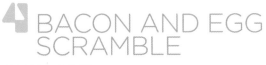

4 BACON AND EGG SCRAMBLE

YOU'LL NEED

2 slices bacon
2 eggs

½ avocado
1 teaspoon chia seeds

HOW TO MAKE IT

1. Cook the bacon according to the package instructions. After flipping, add the eggs to the pan. Cook for 1 minute and then scramble the eggs as the bacon cooks. Cook until the desired consistency is reached. Remove from the pan. Slice the avocado and top the slices with chia seeds. Serve alongside the bacon-and-egg mixture.

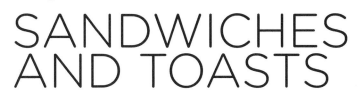

SANDWICHES AND TOASTS

5 AB+J

YOU'LL NEED

2 slices gluten-free bread
½ cup blueberries

2 tablespoons almond butter

HOW TO MAKE IT

1. Toast the bread. Meanwhile, mash the berries into a paste. After the bread is toasted, spread almond butter on the bread, and add the berry spread. Combine into a sandwich.

6 WAFFLE SANDWICH

YOU'LL NEED

1 gluten-free frozen waffle
2 tablespoons peanut butter

½ cup raspberries

HOW TO MAKE IT

1. Cook the waffle according to the package instructions. Spread the peanut butter on the waffle. Add the berries and form the waffle into a sandwich.

7 SLAMMIN' SALMON

YOU'LL NEED

1 gluten-free frozen waffle
½ avocado

Dash of smoked paprika
1 ounce smoked salmon

HOW TO MAKE IT

1. Cook the waffle according to the package instructions. Mash the avocado and smoked paprika. Spread on the waffle. Top with the salmon.

8 AVOCADO NOOCH TOAST

YOU'LL NEED

1 slice gluten-free bread
½ avocado
Red pepper flakes to taste

1 tablespoon nutritional yeast
Pinch of salt

HOW TO MAKE IT

1. Toast the bread. Meanwhile, mash the avocado with red pepper flakes, nutritional yeast, and a pinch of salt. When the toast is done, spread the avocado mixture on top and enjoy.

9 THE LEAN BEAN

YOU'LL NEED

1 gluten-free English muffin
1 teaspoon olive oil
1 egg

¼ cup black beans
¼ sliced avocado
Pinch of cayenne pepper

HOW TO MAKE IT

1. Toast the English muffin. Meanwhile, heat a nonstick frying pan over medium-high heat. Add the olive oil. Crack the eggs into a pan and let cook until the egg white is a bit firm, and then add the beans. Scramble the mixture with a fork in the pan. Cook until the desired consistency is reached. Remove from the heat.

2. Add the mixture between the English muffin halves to make a sandwich. Add the avocado and cayenne (or spices of your choice). Enjoy.

5 GRAB-AND-GO OPTIONS

1 1 Dark Chocolate and Sea Salt Kind Bar **+** 1 handful of blueberries

2 1 scoop vanilla or chocolate plant-based protein powder **+** 1 cup unsweetened almond milk (blended in a shaker bottle)

3 2 hard-boiled eggs **+** 4 strawberries

4 1 Silk Plain Almond Dairy-Free Yogurt Alternative **+** 10 almonds

5 2 Applegate Natural turkey slices **+** an apple

OATMEAL AND CEREALS

10 CRAZY BUSY OATMEAL

YOU'LL NEED

1 cup water
½ cup oatmeal
½ cup almond milk

1 scoop plant-based vanilla or chocolate protein powder (this recipe works best with Kashi, which is easiest to blend)
1 teaspoon chia seeds
½ banana

HOW TO MAKE IT

1. Combine water and oats in a bowl and microwave for 2 minutes. Remove and add almond milk and protein powder. Mix until smooth. Add the chia seeds and banana.

11 MESA SUNRISE
WITH PROTEIN BOOST

YOU'LL NEED

¾ cup Nature's Path Gluten-Free Mesa Sunrise
½ cup almond milk

1 scoop plant-based vanilla or chocolate protein powder (this recipe works best with Kashi, which is easiest to blend)

HOW TO MAKE IT

1. Combine the ingredients in a bowl, stir until powder dissolves, and enjoy.

12 INSTANT CHOCOLATE OATS

YOU'LL NEED

1 cup water
½ cup oatmeal
½ cup almond milk

1 scoop plant-based chocolate
  protein powder
1 teaspoon chocolate chips

HOW TO MAKE IT

1. Combine water and oats in a bowl and microwave for 2 minutes. Remove and add the almond milk and protein powder. Top with chocolate chips.

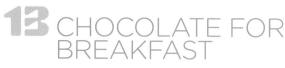

SMOOTHIES AND SMOOTHIE BOWLS

13 CHOCOLATE FOR BREAKFAST

YOU'LL NEED

½ cup frozen blueberries
1½ teaspoon natural,
  no-salt-added almond butter
½ cup unsweetened almond milk

1 scoop chocolate plant-based
  protein powder
Water to blend (optional)

HOW TO MAKE IT

1. Blend the ingredients until smooth and enjoy.

14 LEMON-VANILLA CREME

YOU'LL NEED

½ **lemon,** peeled and seeded
½ **frozen banana**
1 cup spinach
½ cup unsweetened almond milk

1 scoop vanilla plant-based protein
  powder
3 ice cubes
Water to blend (optional)

HOW TO MAKE IT

1. Blend the ingredients until smooth and enjoy.

15 KISS THE KIWI BOWL

YOU'LL NEED

FOR THE SMOOTHIE
Handful of spinach
Almond butter
½ avocado
Maca powder
½ frozen banana
½ regular banana
Squeeze of lime juice
½ cup almond milk

FOR GARNISH
¼ fresh papaya
⅓ kiwi
1 teaspoon bee pollen
Pinch of chia seeds

HOW TO MAKE IT

1. Blend the smoothie ingredients until smooth and then pour into a bowl. Top with the garnishes and serve.

16 BEG FOR CHOCOLATE BOWL

YOU'LL NEED

FOR THE SMOOTHIE
½ frozen banana
1 regular banana
½ cup unsweetened plant-based yogurt
1 teaspoon peanut butter
1 tablespoon cacao powder

FOR GARNISH
3 strawberries
1 tablespoon cacao nibs
Pinch of chia seeds
2 tablespoons pomegranate seeds
1 tablespoon semisweet chocolate chips
1 teaspoon sliced almonds

HOW TO MAKE IT

1. Blend the smoothie ingredients until smooth and then pour into a bowl. Top with the garnishes and serve.

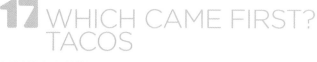

LEFTOVERS FOR BREAKFAST

17 WHICH CAME FIRST? TACOS

YOU'LL NEED

1 teaspoon olive oil

2 eggs

¼ **leftover cooked and sliced chicken breast**

1 corn tortilla

2 tablespoons salsa

Hot sauce, to taste

HOW TO MAKE IT

1. Heat a nonstick frying pan over medium-high heat. Add the olive oil. Crack the eggs into the pan and let cook until the egg whites are a bit firm. Then add chicken and scramble the mixture. Cook until desired consistency is reached. Remove from the heat.

2. Insert the mixture into the corn tortilla to make a breakfast taco. Add the salsa and hot sauce to taste, and enjoy.

18 TURKEY LURKY

YOU'LL NEED

1 teaspoon olive oil
2 eggs
¼ leftover cooked ground turkey

½ cup salsa
Handful of spinach (optional)

HOW TO MAKE IT

1. Heat a nonstick frying pan over medium-high heat. Add the olive oil. Crack the eggs into the pan and add the turkey and salsa. Cook until the eggs are the desired consistency. Remove and serve—over spinach, if you'd like.

19 CHICKEN AND WAFFLE

YOU'LL NEED

1 gluten-free waffle
½ leftover cooked and sliced
    chicken breast

Touch of pure maple syrup

HOW TO MAKE IT

1. Toast the waffle according to the package instructions. Slice the chicken breast. Drizzle a touch of maple syrup onto the waffle and top with the chicken.

20 PEACHY QUINOA

YOU'LL NEED

½ cup leftover cooked quinoa
½ peach, diced

⅓ cup sliced almonds
Touch of unsweetened coconut milk

HOW TO MAKE IT

1. Combine the ingredients together and enjoy.

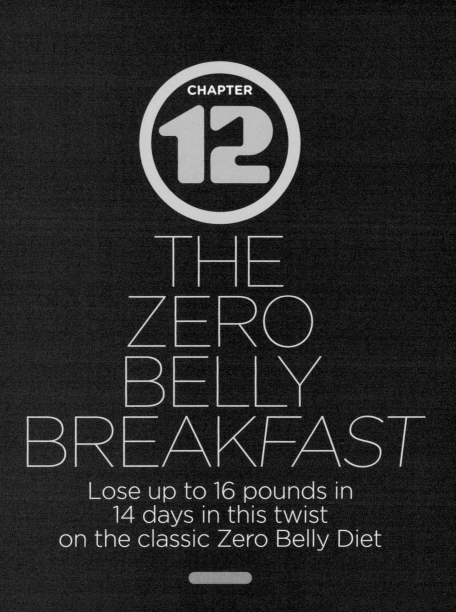

12

THE ZERO BELLY BREAKFAST

Lose up to 16 pounds in
14 days in this twist
on the classic Zero Belly Diet

t's the ultimate trifecta: a smaller waist, a heftier IQ, and a longer, healthier life. And now, science may be on the verge of figuring out one very easy way to achieve them all.

A new study funded by the National Institute on Aging has uncovered a diet plan that can put you on the path to all three—in just days. And you're holding it in your hands.

You see, researchers found that cutting daily calories in half (in the study, for four days every two weeks) reduced biomarkers for aging, diabetes, heart disease, and cancer with no adverse effects. "It isn't a typical diet because it's not something you have to stay on," said lead researcher Valter Longo of the University of Southern California.

They tested the eating plan, called a "fasting mimicking diet" (FMD), on yeast, mice, and humans. Turns out, it doesn't matter what species you are: The results remained consistent across all three groups. The yeast and mice studies showed that the diet increased life span, while a pilot study given to 19 human subjects indicated that the same approach could not only slow the physical and mental aging process but also help slash belly fat accumulation.

The diet "mimics" fasting because you're not cutting out all food. Instead, researchers reduced the individual's caloric intake down to 34 to 54 percent of normal for four consecutive days every two weeks.

Longo believes that for most people, the FMD can be done every three to six months, depending on one's health and body weight. Another study shows that you are more likely to preserve your lean body mass while losing body fat on an alternate-day calorie restriction rather than a continuous low-calorie diet; hunger seems to decrease and satiety increases.

But you don't have to slash calories four days in a row—during a busy workweek—to reap some rewards of fasting. Between shuttling the kids to extracurriculars and fixing family meals, sometimes you just can't block off four days straight.

In this special bonus plan—I call it the Zero Belly BreakFAST—you'll block off every other day instead. Fasting in this pattern leads to a 10-plus-pound weight loss, according to a study out of the University of Illinois. And it may also be beneficial in more extreme cases; obese adults who tried this particular method of intermittent fasting (and also added exercise into the mix) lost weight, fried fat, and slashed bad cholesterol—while boosting good cholesterol—according to research published in the journal *Obesity*. Here's how it works.

THE ZERO BELLY BREAKFAST PLAN

On even-numbered "fast" days, you'll enjoy:

- A Zero Belly Breakfast in the morning
- A Zero Belly Smoothie for lunch
- Another Zero Belly Smoothie for dinner

Which puts you in a negative calorie state.

On odd-numbered days, you'll enjoy:

The meals as detailed in *Zero Belly Diet*—that's three Zero Belly meals, one Zero Belly Smoothie, and one additional Zero Belly snack per day.

All days, limit

- processed foods
- saturated fat
- sugar
- refined grains
- wheat and dairy

All days, maximize the Zero Belly Foods, which include:

- high-phytonutrient fruits and vegetables
- high-fiber, high-protein nuts, legumes, and grains
- monounsaturated and polyunsaturated fats
- omega-3 fatty acids

Alcohol

Limit to one glass of wine per day, but no alcohol on fast days.

Duration

Stick to the schedule for two weeks and see how you feel. You should notice changes after week one!

SECRET WEAPON

LEPTIN, THE HUNGER HORMONE

Fasting at first sounds rough, but the secret is spending your calories on foods that boost your levels of leptin, a hormone that controls hunger. Start your day with a bowl of oats; this breakfast staple is packed with insoluble fiber, which one Canadian study showed can boost levels of leptin.

MAKE THE FAST GO FASTER

To get the most out of your Zero Belly BreakFAST, always remember these three secrets.

Don't resist resistant starch

If you're going on a fast—or dieting—your first instinct might be to avoid all carbs, since they break down quickly in your body and can grow belly fat. But if you choose the right starchy foods, they can actually help you sail through your four days of fasting and trim down in the process. Slightly underripe bananas and white beans should both be on your menu during your fast as they're rich in resistant starch. This type of starch resists digestion (hence, the name) so it passes through the small intestine without being digested. This feeds healthy gut bacteria, leading to prolonged feelings of fullness and more efficient fat oxidation. (Cool weight-loss secret: When you chill pasta, it turns into a resistant starch.)

Hit the hay earlier

Getting enough quality sleep is crucial for hunger regulation and even healthy weight loss. A recent study found subpar sleep could undermine weight loss by as much as 55 percent. Inadequate or broken sleep can throw hunger-regulating hormones out of balance. Ghrelin, the "I'm hungry" hormone, shoots up; leptin, the "I'm full!" hormone, decreases. The result? You're hungrier, grumpier, and you eat more food. Plus, going to bed early and logging a full eight hours a night while you're fasting makes it easier to bypass less than virtuous late-night cravings.

Go back to the well

Drinking enough water will not only fill your stomach and ward off hunger, but it also keeps your energy levels up and your metabolism from dipping while you're eating less. But plain water can get boring, so mix in glasses of water spiked with pieces of fresh fruit and cups of tea.

Eat pure, drink pu-erh

This fermented Chinese tea can literally shrink the size of your fat cells! To discover the brew's fat-crusading powers, Chinese researchers divided rats into five groups and fed them varying diets over a two-month period. In addition to a control group, there was a group given a high-fat diet with no tea supplementation and three additional groups that were fed a high-fat diet with varying doses of pu-erh tea extract. The researchers found that the tea significantly lowered triglyceride concentrations (potentially dangerous fat found in the blood) and belly fat in the high-fat diet groups. Although sipping the tea could have slightly different outcomes in humans, we think these findings are promising enough that it's still well worth your while to fix yourself a steaming hot cup.

FAST ANSWERS

Do I have to count calories on the Zero Belly BreakFAST?

Not if you use Zero Belly recipes. But if you're curious about calories: You need to be in a negative-calorie state in order to lose weight—meaning burning off more calories than you are taking in—so you will be consuming fewer calories than you're probably used to eating.

Are there really no snacks on "fast" days?

You will not have a snack on the "fast" days, so your body can remain in a negative-calorie state. The next day, you will be allowed to have three meals and healthy snacks.

What if I'm super-hungry on my "fast" days?

You might be hungry in the first few days, as you adjust to this schedule. Keep water, green tea, or other calorie-free beverages on hand for when hunger strikes—staying hydrated can help ward off hunger. Studies show, after three days, your body will adjust and your hunger will decrease.

Do I have to eat like this forever?

No. You can go back to normal meals—though keep your meals healthy and Zero Belly approved! —if you feel that you have gotten into your healthy weight range. You can always go back to this alternate-day diet plan when you need a reset.

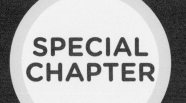

SPECIAL CHAPTER

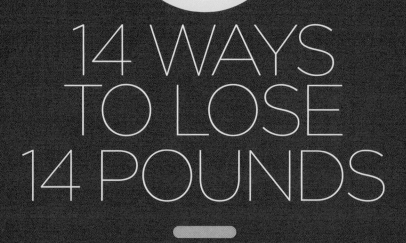

14 WAYS TO LOSE 14 POUNDS

"I can't do this. I can't face another diet."

My friend Kimberly was making yet another series of desperate New Year's weight-loss resolutions.

"Every year, I starve myself for months, I lose maybe five pounds, and by springtime it all comes back," she complained. "What's the point? I'm just destined to be overweight."

"What would you say if I told you that you didn't need to go on a diet for months or even weeks?" I asked Kim. "What if you could lose much of that belly in just 14 days?" Simply making a handful of tweaks to your diet and lifestyle can help improve your gut health, dampen inflammation, turn off your fat genes, and start your body shedding fat—in particular, the fat belly—almost automatically. Here's how.

14 Take a brisk walk before breakfast

Zero Belly Diet panelist Martha Chesler did just this as part of her Zero Belly program, and the results were astonishing. "I saw changes immediately," she reports. In less than six weeks on the program, Martha dropped over 20 pounds and an astonishing 7 inches from her middle by combining the Zero Belly Foods with a pre-breakfast walk.

This easy a.m. ritual works on two levels. First, a recent study found that exposure to sunlight in between the hours of 8 a.m. and noon reduced your risk of weight gain regardless of activity level, caloric intake, or age. Researchers speculate that the morning light synchronizes your metabolism and undercuts your fat genes. And burning calories before you eat means you're exercising in a fasted state—the energy you burn comes right from your fat stores, instead of the food you ate. But what really stunned Martha was the improvement in her heart health. Before starting Zero Belly Diet, Martha's heart rate would typically soar to 112 beats per minute (bpm) within moments of starting her exercise bike workout. "After the first week and a half I could not raise my heart rate over 96 bpm with the same workout. It was great to see change in the mirror, and even better to know good things were happening that I couldn't even see."

13 Grab a nutcracker

Naturally sweet oatmeal recipes in *Zero Belly Diet* were the key to test panelist Isabel Fiolek's dramatic 13-pound weight loss. "I happen to have a big sugar addiction," Isabel admits, "but the recipes have been surprisingly satisfying for my sweet tooth." Isabel also made dramatic health strides: A checkup after her six weeks on Zero Belly Diet revealed she'd dropped her total cholesterol by 25 percent and her blood glucose level by 10 percent.

For an extra boost in your oatmeal, add walnuts. Omega-3 fatty acids, the nutrients that make fatty fish such nutritional champs, play a key role in reducing belly fat storage, all while keeping us full and satisfied. But thankfully you don't have to down an entire fillet or even turn on the stove to reap their stomach-flattening benefits. Just ¼ cup of walnuts packs more than two days' worth of ALA (alpha-linolenic acid), a type of omega-3 fatty acid. And bonus: Walnuts have also been shown to reduce blood pressure and decrease inflammation in the blood vessels during times of stress.

12 Choose red fruit over green

It's the best fruit for weight loss. That means Pink Lady over Granny Smith, watermelon over honeydew, red grapes over green ones. The higher levels of nutrients called flavonoids—particularly anthocyanins, compounds that give red fruits their color—calm the action of fat-storage genes. In fact, red-bellied stone fruits such as plums boast phenolic compounds that have been shown to modulate the expression of fat genes.

11 Make some guacamole

For test panelist June Caron, incorporating fresh produce like avocados was a life-changing lesson from *Zero Belly Diet*. The 55-year-old lost 6 pounds in the first week on the program. "Learning to eat real, chemical-free fresh foods has been the best thing that ever happened to me. I am never hungry. And the weight just keeps coming off!" Glowing skin, healthy nails, and better sleep were Zero Belly bonuses, June said. "I'm well on my way to getting my sexy back. Everyone says I look much younger!"

Avocados are a double-whammy to belly fat. First, they're packed with heart-healthy monounsaturated fats that dim your hunger switches; a study in *Nutrition Journal* found that participants who ate half a fresh avocado with lunch reported a 40 percent decreased desire to eat for hours afterward. Second, unsaturated fats like those found in avocados seem to prevent the storage of belly fat.

10 Pick the right protein

Test panelist Bryan Wilson, a 29-year-old accountant, lost 19 pounds and an astounding 6 inches from his waist in just six weeks on the program, and he attributes his success to the Zero Belly shake recipes in the program. "I love the shakes. I added them to my diet, and almost immediately I lost the bloat," Bryan said. "I'm a sweet craver, and the shakes were an awesome alternative to the bowls and bowls of ice cream I would have had."

Protein drinks are great ways to get a monster dose of belly-busting nutrition into a delicious, simple snack. But most commercial protein shakes are filled with unpronounceable chemicals that can upset our gut health and cause inflammation and bloat. And the high doses of whey used to boost protein levels can amplify the belly-bloating effect. The Zero Belly solution: Try vegan protein, which will give you the same fat-burning, hunger-squelching, muscle-building benefits, without the bloat.

9 Make a note to yourself

Subtle, even subliminal, messages may be more effective at helping us stick to a healthy eating regimen than even ongoing, conscious focus, found a 2015 study in the *Journal of Marketing Research*. The study found that people who receive reinforcing notes urging them to eat healthy were more likely to make smarter choices than those who tried to keep their goals top of mind at all times. Simple reminders—keeping a bowl of nuts on your kitchen counter, for example, or putting reminders into your phone—will keep you on the winning side.

8 Mix up a magic elixir

Start each day by making a large pitcher of "spa water"—that's detox water filled with sliced whole lemons, oranges, or grapefruits—and make a point of sipping your way through at least 8 glasses before bedtime. Citrus fruits are rich in the antioxidant delimonene, a powerful compound found in the peel that stimulates liver enzymes to help flush toxins from the body and gives sluggish bowels a kick, according to the World Health Organization.

7 Make your own trail mix

The three major ingredients of a perfect Zero Belly meal or snack are protein, fiber, and healthy fats, and all three can be found in abundance in a good trail mix. Sadly, most commercial mixes are made with extra oils, salt, and sugar. Mix up your own high-protein snacks from a selection of nuts, seeds, unsweetened dried fruit, and dark chocolate pieces.

Snaxercise

The biggest reason we can't stick to our workouts? No time. Trying to squeeze a trip to the gym, with a shower and change of clothes, into a hectic schedule—especially around the holidays—can make even the most dedicated fitness buff into someone, well, less buff. But scientists in New Zealand recently found that men and women who engaged in three 10-minute exercise "hors d'oeuvres" before breakfast, lunch, and dinner saw lowered blood glucose levels—a fat-busting benefit these folks showed all day long!

The short circuits in *Zero Belly Diet* offer a variety of exercises that blast your core without relying on traditional sit-ups—easy enough to squeeze in before dinner in the comfort of your living room. Within six weeks of incorporating the mini circuits, test panelist Krista Powell lost 25 pounds—and she was finally able to dress in a way that reflected her true sense of style: "I'd avoided wearing high heels because the extra weight made my knees hurt so bad. I can actually wear my heels with confidence and without pain!"

Rethink your supplements

If you're taking lots of vitamins and probiotics each day, you may want to reevaluate your strategy. Increased levels of B vitamins have long been associated with a higher prevalence of obesity and diabetes, perhaps because megadosing triggers our fat genes. A daily multivitamin is probably fine, but don't try to convince yourself that more is better. And a recent study by ConsumerLab.com found that most commercial probiotics have far less healthy bacteria than they claim. Your better bet is to focus on the Zero Belly foods to ensure your belly is getting plenty of love—and your fat genes are being cut off at the pass.

4 Have dark chocolate & berries for dessert

Indulging in delicious food is a core principle of Zero Belly Diet. It was the balanced, "zero sacrifice" approach that helped test panelist Jennie Joshi finally lose her pregnancy weight. In just over a month on Zero Belly Diet, Jennie lost 11 pounds, "and the pregnancy pooch is leaving!" she said. "I couldn't believe I was indulging in dark chocolate—and finally getting results! It's a lifestyle, not a diet. It's easy to stick with, and it makes sense."

It makes scientific sense, also: A recent study found that antioxidants in cocoa prevented laboratory mice from gaining excess weight and actually lowered their blood sugar levels. And another study at Louisiana State University found that gut microbes in our stomach ferment chocolate into heart-healthy, anti-inflammatory compounds that shut down genes linked to insulin resistance and inflammation. Why the berries? The fruit speeds up the fermentation process, leading to an even greater reduction in inflammation and weight.

3 Swap farmed salmon for wild salmon

Lean protein like fish is a great way to fight fat and boost your metabolism. But the farmed salmon you get at the local market might not be the best bet for your belly. The cold-water fish has a well-deserved reputation for packing plenty of heart-healthy omega-3 fatty acids—1,253 mg of the good stuff, and just 114 mg of inflammatory, belly-busting omega-6s. But the farmed variety—and 90 percent of what we eat today is farmed—has a very different story to tell. It packs a whopping 1,900 mg of unhealthy omega-6s.

2 Eat a better peanut butter

Real peanut butter is made with two ingredients: peanuts, and maybe some salt. You already know that peanuts give you belly-slimming monounsaturated fats, tummy-filling fiber, and metabolism-boosting protein. But peanuts have a hidden weapon in their weight-loss utility belt: genistein, a compound that acts directly on the genes for obesity, helping to turn them down and reduce your body's ability to store fat. (Beans and lentils have the same magic ingredient, albeit in slightly less delicious form.) But be careful of the brand you buy: If you see ingredients like sugar, palm oil, or anything you can't pronounce, put it back. They'll undermine any good the peanuts might do.

1 Pregame lunch and dinner with greens

High-volume, low-calorie greens will fill you up, without filling you out. Test panelist Kyle Cambridge says regular salads turbocharged his success: "My wife Stacie and I decided to add salad to each meal, and the pounds started melting off." Kyle lost 25 pounds and four inches in just six weeks on the program. "I even had to buy a new belt!" he said. "But the best was when Stacie came up to me in the kitchen and gave me a hug. She laughed and smiled and said, 'I can wrap my hands around you again.'"

Leafy greens such as collard greens, watercress, kale, and arugula may not be on your everyday list, but they all contain a compound called sulforaphane. This nutrient has been shown to act directly on the genes that determine "adipocyte differentiation"—basically, turning a stem cell into a fat cell. A healthier intake of the compound means a healthier body weight for you. And just a scant teaspoon of vinaigrette will help your body absorb the fat-soluble nutrients.

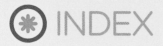

INDEX

Page numbers in *italics* refer to photographs.

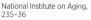